*Losing Weight
for Good*

Lawrence J. Cheskin, M.D., is Director of the
Johns Hopkins Weight Management Center
and Associate Professor at the Johns Hopkins
School of Medicine and the School of Hygiene
and Public Health

Losing Weight for Good

Developing Your Personal Plan of Action

Lawrence J. Cheskin, M.D.

The Johns Hopkins University Press
Baltimore and London

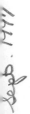

Note to the Reader: This book describes a personal approach to weight loss. It is not intended to take the place of your relationship with your physician or to substitute for medical treatment of obesity. If you are seriously overweight, are out of shape, are over the age of 40, or have a history of medical problems, we recommend that you seek the advice of a physician before beginning a weight loss program.

© 1997 The Johns Hopkins University Press
All rights reserved. Published 1997
Printed in the United States of America on acid-free recycled paper
06 05 04 03 02 01 00 99 98 97   5 4 3 2 1

Chapter 6 was written with Lori W. Wiersema, M.S., R.D., L.D. The Pyramid Tables for Weight Management and the Pyramid Pattern Menus, which appear at the end of this book, were developed by Lori W. Wiersema, M.S., R.D., L.D.

The Johns Hopkins University Press
2715 North Charles Street
Baltimore, Maryland 21218-4319
The Johns Hopkins Press Ltd., London

Library of Congress Cataloging-in-Publication Data will be found at the end of this book.
A catalog record for this book is available from the British Library.

ISBN 0-8018-5499-7

To my wife, Gail Stern,
always an inspiration

Contents

Preface

For the past eight years, the Johns Hopkins Weight Management Center has been providing innovative programs to people who need to lose weight. The treatment programs are unique in several ways.

First, they were developed by professionals at Johns Hopkins, an institution widely regarded as the world's finest in the field of medicine. Second, the treatment programs are based on the latest research in the fields most important to weight management—medicine, behavioral psychology, nutrition, and exercise physiology. Third, and most important, the programs were designed to take into account differences between people.

People who need to lose weight are individuals, with special needs, interests, and goals. Since people gain weight for different reasons, the programs of the Johns Hopkins Weight Management Center start with a careful assessment of the individual by a team of experts—a physician, a behavioral psychologist, a nutritionist, and an exercise physiologist. These experienced team members coordinate their efforts to put together an individualized Plan of Action in consultation with the individual seeking help.

The individualized plan always contains certain key ingredients crucial for lasting success—an attainable goal, an appealing diet, an enjoyable exercise program, and an opportunity to learn about oneself, build self-confidence, and make satisfying changes in lifestyle and attitude.

Now, in this book, for the first time, many of the advantages of a comprehensive, individualized program put together by a team of experts are available to the individual who needs to lose weight and wishes to do it effectively, on his or her own. What I have done is carefully translate the elements of this comprehensive program, to guide the reader, step by step, through a self-assessment process leading to selection of just those aspects of the program which will address his or her specific needs. By following these steps, the reader develops his or her own Personal Plan, one that takes into account individual needs and focuses attention on the areas that need it most—a plan that will help the reader not just to lose weight now but to keep it off into the next millennium.

As I write this Preface, I am participating in the annual meeting of the North American Association for the Study of Obesity. I am struck by the consensus that is building among this distinguished group of physicians and scientists that an individualized approach offers the best chance of success to people who are struggling to control their weight. This is precisely the theme of this book.

Over a third of Americans are now overweight, up from a quarter only a decade or so ago. Almost half the adult U.S. population has tried to lose weight in the past year. Books and programs that attempt to force everyone into the same treatment mold can succeed only for those who fit the mold. This book is different. Instead of the usual platitudes and formulaic advice, it presents a case for individualized treatment which takes into account the many different paths to becoming overweight. A 40-year-old recently divorced woman who is low on self-esteem and compulsively overeats, and a 55-year-old man who runs his own business and loves big home-cooked meals and beer, may both be 50 pounds overweight, but for entirely different reasons. Pick up the usual diet book, and you will find both these people being advised to cut fat from their diets and to exercise more. Such advice does nothing to get at the underlying problems and invites more frustration and despair, emotions all too familiar to people who have tried and repeatedly failed to get their weight under control using the one-diet-fits-all approach.

Instead of false promises, this book offers hope and reassurance tempered by realism and sound advice. The basic message is this: You do not need to change everything about yourself and your life to lose weight and keep it off. You do need to identify your specific problem areas and find creative, individualized solutions. This book will help you create your own Personal Plan of Action. It is a tool combining assessment, education, and practical advice that will enable you to meet your problem head on—and even enjoy yourself along the way.

Acknowledgments

In a work like this, there are many contributors and kinds of contributions. I would like to thank my son, Eric, for his devotion and understanding when the pressures of work and deadlines interfered with our time together; my parents, Al and Greta Cheskin, for instilling their belief that no goal is impossible, including writing a book; and my wife, Gail Stern, for her ideas, her help, and her unwavering support.

The inspiration for this book arose, of course, from the many people who have come to the Johns Hopkins Weight Management Center to seek help managing a weight problem. Through their example I have learned much about the value of persistence and commitment.

Before the idea for this book could even be conceived, though, the Johns Hopkins Weight Management Center had to exist. Its start in 1990 was made possible by a number of people: my department chairman, Dr. Phil Zieve, whose wisdom and support have often enabled me to exceed even his expectations; Dr. Phil Katz, who graciously encouraged me to take on the task of starting a weight management program at Johns Hopkins; Mr. Ron Peterson, who took a chance and provided the support of the Johns Hopkins Bayview Medical Center from the very start; Dr. Bill Vitale, whose generosity and experience sustained us through the crucial formative years; Dr. Marvin Schuster, my division chief, who allowed me to devote the time necessary to ensure the success of the Johns Hopkins Weight Management Center; and, of course, the staff of the program, most of whom are still with me, helping people in need.

The genesis of this book was aided greatly by my friend Nan Heneson. Judy Waranch also provided helpful advice. The writing process was a new experience for me. I am indebted to my editor at the Johns Hopkins University Press, Jackie Wehmueller, for having the confidence in me to suggest that I write this book, and for her patience and wise advice while shepherding me ably (and persistently) through the writing. Also at the Press, my heartfelt thanks to Carol Ehrlich, who expertly handled the later stages of the editorial process, and Lynn Cook, who carefully reviewed each chapter, providing a number of excellent suggestions. Expert review of the manuscript was also kindly provided by Dr. David Allison of the New York Obesity Research Center; Dr. Philip Eichling, medical director of Canyon Ranch, provided helpful suggestions on Chapter 2.

My thanks to Jean Edsall and Stacey Bennett for typing the manuscript, and to Debbie Tourtlotte for her timely assistance with the index.

A special thanks to Lori Wiersema, associate director for nutrition at the Johns Hopkins Weight Management Center, who taught me much of what I know about weight management and nutrition and who contributed the material for Chapter 6 and the food tables and menus.

I am grateful to Dr. Susan Bartlett, associate director for clinical psychology at the Johns Hopkins Weight Management Center, who reviewed the behavioral material in her usual thorough manner, and to Dr. Ross Andersen, associate director for exercise physiology, who did likewise for exercise material. I appreciate the research and comments I received from Dr. Kevin Fontaine, associate director for research psychology at the center. If I have accomplished anything of value in writing this book, I must also credit my colleagues Drs. Ben Caballero, Reubin Andres, and Ivan Barofsky.

Without these individuals, there would have been no book. I am glad to have the chance to acknowledge their contributions and to express my appreciation.

*Losing Weight
for Good*

ONE

Why Lose Weight?

As you drive along the highway, your car radio blares, "You can lose weight now! Call now for your no-cost, no-obligation introduction!" The billboards you pass along the way feature svelte people enjoying all the good things in life. Even the people in the fast food ads seem to have gained nary an ounce from consuming their food of choice.

Is this a true representation of reality, or is this a treacherous highway—and not because of icy roads? Clearly, there's something going on here. For one thing, most people cannot indulge regularly in fast food and stay thin. Do we ignore both the fantasy billboards and the radio commercial and drive blindly on, or do we slow down and think about this issue? If we don't look like the people in the ads, do we care? Or is it okay to be overweight?

The answer is that we do care. Recent medical research shows that being moderately to severely overweight can take years away from your life. And we can all name ways in which being overweight can diminish our quality of life as well. The consequences of being overweight, though extremely variable, fall into two general categories: medical and social.

Down through history, being heavy was more often considered a positive attribute than a negative one. Only those who were well off could afford to eat more than they needed and to avoid physical labor. Also, people did not live long enough to make the health risks of being obese apparent, so the "down side" was minimal. In terms of aesthetics, art had always favored the rotund model. Only in the past fifty years (and, indeed, only in certain cultures) has thinness become a societal ideal.

It is now widely accepted that being moderately to seriously overweight is a risk to your health. More precisely, having an excess of body fat is the risk. People who are overweight for their height are sometimes athletic or engage in a lot of strenuous physical labor. This often results in a muscular, "overweight," but not overfat, person. If you are reading this book, this is probably not your situation. You are probably someone who has tried fad diets and weight-loss programs before, with limited success. You may be looking for help developing a rational, long-term approach to weight loss that involves permanent lifestyle changes. If so, you've come to the right place.

In this book, I will share with you the benefits of my experience as a physician and scientist with the Johns Hopkins Weight Management Center. The plan I describe is the Personal Plan of Action. I will carefully and honestly describe methods that have helped hundreds of other people lose weight, while at the same time offering some advice that, if followed, can improve your health and psychological well-being, whether you lose weight or not. First, let's consider some important aspects of gaining and losing weight.

The way excess fatty tissue is *distributed* in the body is now believed to be at least as important as the *amount* of excess fat in determining a person's health risk. Are you an "apple" or a "pear" when it comes to body fat? Excess fat deposited around the middle (the apple figure) is much riskier in terms of fostering heart disease than an equal amount of excess fat around the hips, thighs, or buttocks (the pear figure). Fortunately, fat around the middle comes off first and most readily when you lose weight. Fat concentrated in the lower body, as many have learned the hard way, is remarkably resistant to modest weight loss.

Being severely overweight is a risk factor for a host of medical problems. Most common: high blood pressure, high cholesterol, heart disease, stroke, and diabetes. Other common medical problems, like bone and joint diseases such as arthritis, are made worse when the body is subjected to the strain of carrying around excess weight.

For some people the medical advantages of losing weight are the most important, particularly if the person has developed a health problem such as heart disease, high cholesterol, or diabetes. There is uncertainty and disagreement, however, among experts about the health risks associated with slight to moderate degrees of overweight. While controversy has arisen about the risks of small degrees of excess body fat, there is probably little excess risk of disease for people who are within 20 percent of their "ideal" body weight, and only modest increases in risk of disease and premature death for people who are 20-40 percent over "ideal." For people who are more than 40 percent above "ideal" weight, there is clearly an excess risk of

TABLE 1.1 MEDICAL RISKS OF EXCESS BODY FAT

Non-insulin dependent diabetes mellitus
Hypertension
Coronary artery disease
Hyperlipidemia (high cholesterol)
Strokes
Cancer (endometrial, post-menopausal, breast, colorectal)
Sleep apnea
Gallbladder disease
Gastroesophageal reflux disease (heartburn)
Fatty liver
Osteoarthritis
Gout
Infertility
Thromboembolism (blood clots)

Source: Adapted from Lawrence J. Cheskin, M.D., "Obesity," in *Current Therapy in Gastroenterology and Liver Disease,* 4th ed., ed. Theodore M. Bayless (St. Louis: Mosby Year Book, 1994).

both illness and early death. On the other hand, excess abdominal fat, even when overall weight for height is normal, can increase health risks. (A table showing "ideal" body weight is included in Chapter 6.)

For most people who want to lose weight, though, medical concerns are not foremost. And even for those with medical conditions, the real payoff in losing weight is not so much in improving disease states as in *feeling* better. Many people who have lost weight through the Johns Hopkins Weight Management Center are pleased, for example, that their cholesterol is lower. But more tangible and infinitely more satisfying is the fact that, as 48-year-old Alice said, "I can walk up a flight or two of stairs and not feel like collapsing. I don't get tired so easily anymore. I have so much more energy for doing the things I couldn't do before."

Unfortunately, there is more to the issue of what a desirable weight is in our society than health. The social and emotional consequences of being overweight are enormous. Our society fosters widespread prejudice against the obese, even job discrimination and economic hardship. This prejudice begins at an early age. One study showed pictures of obese and not obese children to a group of seven-year-old boys and girls and asked them to describe the pictures. Even at age seven, children characterized their obese peers as lazy, stupid, and ugly compared with the non-obese children pictured. Sadly, the prejudice is so pervasive that even people who are obese may endorse these negative views about others who are obese. Perhaps the worst consequence of all is how such people must then feel about themselves.

Although many obese people have been tremendously successful in all spheres of life, and many have a positive self-image, it is common for overweight people to have low self-esteem, even clinical depression. It is also remarkably common for obese women seeking treatment at the Johns Hopkins Weight Management Center to have suffered childhood sexual abuse. Such women may unconsciously have gained weight in part to avoid abuse, and have an unspoken fear of losing weight. Even for people who have much less dramatic reasons for their weight problem, the social consequences are usually considered very important, and highly motivating for the individual desiring to lose weight.

The psychosocial consequences of being obese, I believe, are the saddest. I say this because prejudice against people because of their weight is, like other prejudices, grossly unfair and undeserved. Unlike other groups of individuals who suffer from the effects of prejudice in our culture, the obese really don't have an organized peer group to share their burden. The victim of racial or religious prejudice is generally surrounded by supportive members of a peer group who have been hurt by the same prejudice. The obese person usually suffers alone, in silence.

A person can rail against the injustices of our society, participate in organized support groups, and join political lobbies for the obese, but these activities are unlikely to solve that person's weight problem, and society's prejudices are unlikely to disappear in our lifetime. Nevertheless, it is not up to society to convince someone to lose weight. Instead, it is up to each individual to decide for himself or herself. Critical in this process of deciding to lose weight is not to let societal or family pressures take on too much importance. This can happen in at least two entirely different ways—both very common, and both ultimately self-defeating.

First, you may make the mistake of deciding not to lose weight because you resent the unfair pressure to do so by friends, family, or society. This falls in the category of "How I bit off my nose to spite my face."

Second, you may indeed decide to lose weight, not because you are convinced of the personal benefits to be derived from this action, but because someone else wants you to lose weight, or you are expecting the world to treat you better. While doing it for someone else can be motivating in the short run, there is bound to be some resentment of having to suffer the deprivation that losing weight may entail. This lack of true self-motivation to change is likely to make the process more difficult than it need be, and the effort ultimately less likely to succeed.

The better approach is to resolve, if you are to do it at all, to do it for *you*. Yes, there will be external pressures influencing your actions, but they need to be put in the background. If you remind yourself regularly of the reasons *you* wish to lose weight, you will enhance your resolve and your ability to stick to your program.

A word about heredity and obesity. You may have read in the newspapers or heard on TV that several genes have been discovered which influence body weight and metabolism (leptin, GLP-1, and so on). It is certainly true that genetic factors play a role in who becomes overweight, and that we are learning more and more about these factors. In all likelihood, however, these new discoveries will have little or no impact on how we maintain a healthy body weight in the foreseeable future. In fact, although genetic factors may be important, they can't explain the last decade's rise in the proportion of people in the United States who are overweight, from 1 out of every 4 people to 1 out of 3. Our genes have not changed for the worse. Our habits have.

Let me also address the anti-diet backlash, which has been in vogue recently. I am referring to the highly publicized view that diets don't work, that you are better off either living with excess weight or, if you must lose weight, doing so at a rate not to exceed half a pound per week. The fact is that there are numerous examples of abuse and exploitation foisted on a gullible public by the "diet industry." In other words, many "diets" *don't* work. Also, it is clear from various studies that the long-term success of most diet programs is poor. For people who attend formal treatment programs, the available evidence is that only about 5 to 15 percent of those who lose weight will succeed in keeping most of it off five years down the road. For these people diets work, but not for very long.

While these statistics are discouraging when viewed in isolation, it is more helpful to view them in perspective. Let's see whether they can teach us something about how to become members of the "10 percent club"—those who succeed in the long run.

First, it is important to recognize that most published research studies report on the experience of a selected subset of people trying to lose weight. Studies almost always involve people who are referred by their doctors to university weight loss clinics. Such people are often severely obese, poor, and more likely to suffer from depression and other emotional problems. Generally such people are less likely to have the high self-esteem and other resources which are helpful in achieving and maintaining weight loss. What's encouraging is one recent study which says that many people are a lot more successful than the statistics imply. (This is what I think, too.) In one of the largest studies ever carried out, *Consumer Reports* surveyed 95,000 of its readers in 1992 about their dieting habits and success. The survey was completely anonymous, so people had little incentive to lie. Surprisingly, in light of all the dismal pronouncements of experts and the statistics, 4 out of 5 readers had dieted *on their own,* without the help of a weight loss center, and had better results, over the long run, than people in the previous studies on weight loss at formal programs. These people lost an average of 10 pounds. Most importantly, they were more satisfied with their ability to keep the weight off than were people who lost weight through formal programs. A respectable 25 percent of those surveyed were able to keep an average of 70 percent of the weight they had lost off two or more years later, *on their own.* *Consumer Reports* concluded, "The changes they made on their own may have been easier to sustain than the more artificial changes imposed by an outside program." These people are probably much more typical of people who have tried to lose weight than people participating in formal research studies. And the good news is, their success rate is much better!

Although these new statistics are still not as good as we would like, they compare favorably to the long-term success people have in controlling other types of habits, such as cigarette smoking and alcohol and drug abuse. Lest you assume that it is much harder to quit smoking or drinking than to lose weight because smoking and drinking are true addictions, consider this. While the initial stages of going "cold turkey" off of addicting substances are quite unpleasant, we can live quite well without touching another cigarette or drink for the rest of our lives. With overeating, we must learn to deal with the things that get us into trouble every day. There is no escaping food.

Despite this, many people do succeed at losing weight, feeling better, and keeping the weight off. I see them every day at the Johns Hopkins Weight Management Center.

What distinguishes people who do succeed from those who succeed only temporarily or not at all? Although there is no magic formula for success, we do know some things about the typical success stories. People who succeed in achieving and maintaining a desirable goal weight tend to have certain coping skills which keep them on track. These skills are not innate or inherited. *They can be taught, and they can be learned.* The focus of this book is on teaching you the skills that can help you to reach your goals. The following chapters will help you acquire these skills and develop your Personal Plan of Action.

- Getting yourself ready for the challenge of change
- Learning how to assess your needs and develop an individualized Personal Plan of Action involving a diet, increased physical activity, and behavior change
- Setting attainable goals for yourself
- Developing a reliable support system
- Building maintenance skills from the outset
- Becoming invested in your goals
- Taking advantage of the gradual change technique
- Keeping records to keep you on track
- Learning how to make the process of change enjoyable
- Learning how to build flexibility into your Plan

All the best motivations in the world will get you nowhere without a sensible plan designed for your needs. You will design such a plan in Chapter 4. Before that, we need to explore in greater detail your specific motivations and assess your stage of readiness to proceed. That's what the next chapter, "Getting Ready," is all about.

TWO

Getting Ready

You know the scenario. You are all fired up about a new diet. Without hesitation, you join the latest diet program or buy the latest diet book, certain that it will work. You buy or prepare the special food, skim through the directions, and start with the very next meal. It is April 20.

By April 26, not even a whole week, you can hardly believe it. You have lost 2½ pounds! Not only that, if the truth be known, you "cheated" a little on the food, but made up for it by doing lots of extra exercise. Now you're really fired up. Trying to lose weight even faster, you increase your exercise time. You start feeling hungrier, so stray further from the diet, but figure that exercise is the key, anyway. It's May 3, and you've lost (only) another ¾ pound. You are disappointed, especially since you have been working so hard, but you vow to press on. Things come up in the following week which occupy a lot of your time—a project is due at work, relatives visit from out of town. You are not able to stick with the daily exercise or the diet.

It's May 10, and you've regained a pound and a half. That really hurts. The new diet does not seem as miraculous as you thought it was. You tell yourself you will get back on track in a couple of weeks, when you expect your schedule to clear up a bit.

Your schedule does clear up, but you are no longer as motivated as you were when it seemed so easy. The new diet and exercise program you started with such enthusiasm a short month ago is now over, and soon forgotten.

What happened?

You started out very confident. You thought you were ready this time, but the diet still didn't work for long. The truth, probably, is that *you were not ready*. Mere desire is a poor substitute for *planned readiness*. Desire to change is a necessary prerequisite to lasting weight loss, but it is only one component of readiness—and surely the most fickle. Desire can be very strong but usually doesn't last long. Inevitably, passion fades, and the real world intrudes on our desires. Is there a way to overcome this?

This chapter will help you assess and improve your state of readiness for making the changes in your lifestyle which will enable you to achieve long-lasting success in losing weight. You will learn the components and stages of true readiness. You will then apply this knowledge to understanding *your* personal motivators and learn what tends to interfere with *your* making an effective commitment to permanent change. Finally, you will learn how to set up the conditions that will maximize your readiness and be most conducive to long-term success. Once you've done these things you will be ready to begin to develop your Personal Plan of Action, as described in later chapters.

So, what is this all-important thing we call readiness? Some people call it motivation, but it is more than that. Readiness can be understood as having two dimensions, *commitment* and *sustainability*. Commitment can be divided into two components, short-term readiness and long-term readiness. *Short-term readiness* is the urge, the passion to begin immediately. *Long-term readiness* is your conviction that permanent change is necessary and attainable. The first is important in getting started; the second is critical for completing the job. Unfortunately, these two components of commitment are often out of sync. People most commonly have an abundance of short-term readiness and a shortage of long-term conviction. We will see how to get these two factors more in tune with each other in this chapter and again in Chapter 4. The second dimension of readiness is *sustainability,* being able to remain ready and willing to make long-term changes in your lifestyle until you have reached your goal and beyond.

Research by Drs. James Prochaska, Carlo DiClemente, and others has identified six stages in the behavior change process. They are: precontemplation, contemplation, preparation, action, maintenance, and termination. Because most people have difficulty *maintaining* their weight loss, the Personal Plan approach to weight loss stops with five stages of change and ignores the termination stage. The most successful maintainers of weight loss are those who recognize that they are always at some risk of regaining their lost weight and maintain a moderate degree of vigilance. In my opinion, the termination stage inappropriately allows you to ignore the problem, and to assume it is permanently solved. It is safest to assume that you will need to be in a maintenance stage forever after weight loss.

The person in the precontemplation stage is someone who, if he or she has a weight problem, either is unaware of it, or is aware but does not wish to change anything in the near future (six months is often used to define near future). If you are reading this, you clearly have gone beyond the precontemplation stage, but you may have spent years dwelling in this stage in the past. A word of caution. If you know people who fit this description, it is unwise to push them to lose weight. The effort will be fruitless, and may damage your relationship with them. They must progress willingly, and on their own, to a later point in the change process.

The contemplation stage describes a person who is aware of a problem and wishes to do something about it sometime in the next six months, but not right now. You may well be at this stage if you are reading this book. Reading at least parts of this book will help you move to the next stage of change, the preparation stage.

The preparation stage describes a person who is aware of the problem, may have thought about taking action in the past, and has now decided to prepare for action during (at most) the next month. This is the ideal stage to be in while reading this book. If you are at this stage, you will be ready to develop a Personal Plan and move directly to the action stage in a state of planned readiness.

The action stage is self-explanatory. It describes a person who is in the midst of change; in this case, someone who has formulated a plan that addresses his or her individual needs, and is actively carrying it out.

As demonstrated by the story that opened this chapter, not all action stages have an equal likelihood of succeeding. Careful preparation, as can be accomplished through developing a Personal Plan, will enhance your chance of both short-term and long-term success.

How long the action stage lasts is not fixed, but varies from person to person. For making diet- and exercise-related behavior changes, a typical period of action is three to six months. During this stage the new behaviors are practiced and perfected. Active weight loss is occurring.

Being in the action stage does not require that the new habits be carried out consistently every single day. The thing that determines whether a person is in the action stage is whether he or she gets back on the horse after a fall. We learn from our missteps when in the action stage, and use the experience to adjust our Personal Plan to take advantage of the information provided by them.

The action stage can end in one of three ways: frustration, apparent success, or true success. Frustration results when the actions undertaken fail to achieve the change, either because we were unable to carry them out or because they were insufficient for our purposes in the first place. (To avoid this disappointment, it is important to select reasonable goals and design appropriate steps to achieve these goals; see Chapter 4.) Apparent success results when we achieve the short-term goal of weight loss, but fail to achieve consistent behavior-change goals. True success is when we end the action stage having achieved both a reasonable weight and sustainable behavior changes.

The maintenance stage describes a person who has ended an action stage and is now faced with the difficult task of consolidating the temporary changes in behavior made in the action stage into long-term habits. This is undoubtedly the most important stage. It makes little sense to lose weight and rapidly regain it. Such "yo-yoing" may even be unhealthful (although scientists are not sure about this at this time).

How can you successfully keep yourself in the maintenance stage and not regain weight? The answer depends in part on individual factors. These are discussed in detail in Chapter 4, "Developing Your Personal Plan," and Chapter 8, "Keeping It Off." In general, studies have shown that successful maintainers are much more likely than unsuccessful maintainers to continue to monitor what they eat, to continue to exercise, and to have devised a personal eating plan.

The maintenance stage is best viewed as lasting for the rest of your days. This is the only safeguard against relapse that I know of, and it is well worth the effort. Indeed, the longer you continue to live with the changes in lifestyle you initiated in the action stage, the easier it should become to make these changes a permanent part of your life. Eating right and staying physically active can become "good" habits, ones that are every bit as durable as the "bad" habits they have replaced.

What Stage of Readiness Are You In?

Now you know what you need to know in order to determine your personal stage of readiness for the changes ahead. From the descriptions you just read, decide whether you are in precontemplation, contemplation, preparation, action, or maintenance. Fill in the blank: I am in the _____ stage of behavior change.

Are You a Contemplator or Precontemplator?

If you described yourself as being at the contemplation or precontemplation stages, it would be a good idea for you to reread Chapter 1, "Why Lose Weight?" and then make yourself a Personal Balance Sheet like the one below. A balance sheet is simply a list of pros and cons, reasons that you have for wanting to lose weight, balanced against the reasons you do not want to lose weight. Here is a sample Personal Balance Sheet for Aaron, a 48-year-old architect who is 5'9" tall and weighs 218 pounds:

AARON'S PERSONAL BALANCE SHEET
To Lose or Not to Lose . . .

Pros	Cons
Improve health; reduce high blood pressure	Too much trouble
Feel less tired with exertion	Don't want to give up ice cream, etc.
Look better	Hate feeling hungry
Get to buy new clothes	Diet food doesn't taste good

Drawing up a Personal Balance Sheet will put before you a summary of your current situation. It may enable you to see that the reasons for losing are more persuasive than you had imagined, and clearly outweigh the cons. But it may reveal that you have some more work to do before you are really ready to move to the preparation stage.

Aaron's balance sheet reveals some problems and conceals some others. For example, in order for Aaron to succeed, his wife must be supportive of and participate in his Personal Plan—but Aaron's wife doesn't appear in Aaron's balance sheet. Also, Aaron's list of pros are so vague that they could apply to anyone. They may not be strong enough motivators for long-term readiness.

The same pros and cons on a balance sheet will yield completely different decisions for different people, depending upon how important each factor is for the individual. You might read Aaron's cons and say, "It's not going to be that much trouble" or "I can give up ice cream." But for Aaron, as it turned out, "It's too much trouble," combined with the vagueness of the reasons on the "pro" side, were enough to terminate his weight loss attempt. When someone is not convinced of the benefits of making a commitment to losing weight, any effort can be "too much trouble."

The Personal Balance Sheet can be very helpful to someone who is on the fence between precontemplation and contemplation. It can also help you if you are just getting started. It should be saved and updated each month for the duration of your weight loss program, right up through the action stage and beyond. This will remind you of old and new reasons that you have for losing weight, and it can help to keep you on track during maintenance.

Preparing for Change?

If you described yourself as being at the preparation stage, you are probably in the best position to get the full benefit of the suggestions in this book. You, too, should write out a Personal Balance Sheet to remind yourself of the good reasons you have for committing to losing weight and keeping it off.

Ready for Action?

If you described yourself as being in the midst of an action stage, this is as good a time as any to take stock of your goals, the reasons you have undertaken this action (by making a Personal Balance Sheet), and the means you have chosen to reach your goals. I suggest you proceed from this chapter directly to Chapter 4. In this way, you can formalize the actions you have initiated, and make certain that your actions are both consistent with your goals and contain all the key ingredients that will give you the best chance of both short-term and long-term success. The effort you put into this reassessment and specific planning will be rewarded with renewed commitment to your goals and a higher likelihood of achieving them.

Maintaining the Status Quo?

If you described yourself as being at the maintenance stage, congratulations! You have achieved at least initial success in conquering a weight problem. Not everyone is able to get this far. In addition, you should take credit for recognizing how important it is to pay attention to the maintenance stage, and not assume that the problem is solved once you've lost weight. To help you stay at your weight and behavior goals (you guessed it), make a Personal Balance Sheet. List the benefits you have realized in losing weight and keeping it off (both health benefits and personal benefits) in the "pro" column, and the disadvantages of losing weight and keeping it off in the "con" column. If you are having difficulty coming up with "cons" that are important to you, this is a very positive sign. If your "cons" include having to eat a healthful diet and remain physically active, this may be a warning sign that you have only committed to short-term weight control, and are at high risk of regaining weight. If so, you may benefit from reassessing your reasons for losing weight and reminding yourself that temporary weight loss is probably not what you really want or need. In either case, if you are in the maintenance stage, you can benefit in particular from reading chapters 5, 6, 7, and 8 of this book.

Assessing Your Degree of Readiness

What would you say is the degree or intensity of your short-term readiness (urge) and long-term readiness (commitment)? Rate these on a scale from 1 to 10, 1 being not at all ready or committed, 5 being a moderate level of readiness or commitment, and 10 being the most ready or committed you can imagine yourself feeling.

Fill in the number that describes the strength of your short-term readiness and long-term readiness:

My short-term readiness: _____

My long-term readiness: _____

Compare the two numbers you wrote down. It's not unusual for the first number to be larger than the second, because people are often more ready to commit in the short term than in the long term, especially when the long-term results have been disappointing when they have tried to lose weight in the past. If this is true for you, then this time around you'll want to make sure that the action stage is rewarding (to help motivate you for the maintenance stage) as well as smoothly integrated with the maintenance stage, so that the maintenance stage is a natural extension of the action stage.

Look at your numbers again. If you rated your depth of commitment at 5 or lower, it is important to ask yourself what's holding you up. What specific doubts do you have, and where are they coming from? Any doubts or hesitation can limit your ability to succeed, so you'll want to identify them and deal with them before you begin. The following twelve questions will help you do this. The discussion that follows the questions will help you explore and address *your* issues before beginning the action stage.

1. What is your weight history?
   A. I've always been heavy, since childhood.
   B. I've been heavy since my teens or twenties.
   C. I've gained weight slowly over many years.
   D. I've gained weight mostly in the last year or two.
2. Are there specific factors that have contributed to your weight gain?
   A. Quitting cigarettes.
   B. Failure to return to prepregnancy weight after childbirth.
   C. Change in physical activity level (job change, retirement, illness).
   D. Depression.
   E. Change in appetite related to medications.
   F. None of the above.
3. Are you undergoing a lot of life changes or stresses at this time? Place a check mark next to the changes that are going on in your life now or that have taken place in the past year.
   ___Marriage, divorce, separation, or breakup of a long-term relationship.
   ___Death or dying of a loved one.
   ___Job change, job loss, or promotion.
   ___Beginning or end of school.
   ___Personal serious illness or injury.
   ___Change in residence.
   ___Other major stresses.
4. What are your main reasons for wanting to lose weight? (Check as many or as few as you wish.)
   ___To improve my appearance.
   ___To improve my health or reduce my risk of medical problems.
   ___To improve my energy level and exercise tolerance.
   ___To avoid the embarrassment of being overweight.
   ___To please someone important to me.
   ___To _____.
   (Fill in the blank.)

5. Please rank, in order of importance from 1 to 6, whom you would like to lose weight for.
   ___ Spouse or significant other.
   ___ Potential significant others.
   ___ Family/children/parents.
   ___ Friends.
   ___ Strangers/societal pressures.
   ___ Myself, independent of others' wishes.

6. How much weight do you wish to lose?
   A. I wish to lose enough weight to get to my ideal body weight or less.
   B. I wish to lose enough to get most of the way to my ideal body weight, but not that far.
   C. I wish to lose just enough to feel more comfortable or reduce my risk of medical problems, even if I am still moderately overweight.

7. How much have you dieted in the past?
   A. I've never really dieted before.
   B. I've dieted one to a few times before.
   C. I've dieted four or more times before.

8. If you have previously dieted, what was the typical outcome in the short run?
   A. I reached my goal.
   B. I got at least halfway to my goal.
   C. I got less than halfway to my goal.

9. If you have previously dieted, what was the long-term outcome?
   A. I kept off most of the weight for many years.
   B. I regained the weight after keeping most of it off for two or more years.
   C. I regained the weight after keeping most of it off for fewer less than two years.

10. Which statement describes how you believe you will behave *while* dieting?
    A. I will likely have a very hard time adhering to my plan.
    B. I will likely be spotty in adhering to my plan—some good days, some bad days.
    C. I will likely be consistently compliant with my plan.

11. Which statement describes how you believe you will behave after the active dieting phase has been completed?
    A. I will likely go right back to old habits as soon as I've met my weight loss goal.

B. I will likely start out with good habits, then slowly revert to the old habits.

C. I will likely maintain the good new habits for a long time.

12. What factors will play an important role in preventing you from successfully completing a weight loss plan? (Check as many or as few as you wish.)

___Lack of time.

___Lack of physical resources (money, exercise equipment, etc.).

___Lack of motivation.

___Lack of support from spouse, family, or others.

___Major stressful event(s) intrude (change in job, residence, relationships, etc.).

___Need to lose weight becomes less important (for example, illness improves, special event like a wedding is over).

Discussion: Preparing for a Lasting Change

Simply reading through your answers to these twelve questions will give you some quick ideas about what's inspiring you to lose weight—and what might possibly be getting in your way. In what follows, I discuss the significance of the various answers to these questions. You may want to read the discussions pertaining to your answers first. Then read about the other answers, because even though you didn't choose these answers, some of them may be playing a hidden role in your life. Being aware of all the possible responses will make it easier for you to recognize issues in your own life when they crop up during or after the action stage of your Personal Plan.

1. WHAT IS YOUR WEIGHT HISTORY?

A. Only about one out of five people who are overweight as adults experienced childhood onset of weight problems. On the other hand, about four out of five people who were heavy as children continue to have weight problems as adults. People in this category very frequently have an inherited component to their weight problem. Also, obesity in childhood causes increases in the number of fat cells in the body. These cells can never be lost, only reduced in size. Because of this, some researchers believe that childhood-onset obesity is a particularly difficult kind of weight problem to control.

Your experience on past diets may well cause you to agree with this assessment. Although it may, indeed, be more difficult for those with childhood-onset obesity to lose weight and keep it off, the consequences of being overweight are probably more damaging, both medically and in terms of self-esteem, than for those with adult-onset obesity.

Also—and this is very relevant to the aim of enhancing readiness— there is sometimes a tendency to believe that if you have had a problem since childhood, there is no use in trying to do anything about it. This is unproductive thinking. To have the best chance of success, you must recognize the difficulties but consciously banish negative beliefs by replacing them with positive beliefs through learning. First, and foremost, it is simply not true. Many people with lifelong weight problems can and do overcome them. The story at the end of this chapter may be particularly helpful because it emphasizes that change is possible only if you believe in your ability to change.

B. Onset of weight problems in the teens or twenties is a very common pattern. If you are still in this age group, take heart. Your eating patterns have not been entrenched for very long, and are therefore more adaptable to change. In addition, you are likely to have a greater capacity for physical activity to help you maintain a lower weight once you reach it.

C. Slow, subtle weight gain over a period of many years is so common that some recent weight tables adjust recommended weights for age. It is controversial whether weight gain with age in average amounts (typically a pound or less per year) is harmful to your health. Changes in body composition, and decreased physical activity (in the face of undiminished food consumption) probably account for this gradual weight gain in most cases. Many men and some women tend to pack these extra pounds around the abdomen. If this is the case for you, it is especially important to lose this abdominal fat, because it is associated with a high risk of cardiovascular disease and diabetes (as discussed in Chapter 1).

D. If you have gained a lot of weight only in the past couple of years, you may be fortunate. This probably means that your heredity, food choices, or physical activity have protected you in the past from weight gain. Thus, a specific new factor is probably causing the relatively sudden change in weight you have experienced. Specific factors are often easier to treat than the lifelong habits so often responsible for weight problems. Various specific factors are discussed next.

2. ARE THERE SPECIFIC FACTORS THAT HAVE CONTRIBUTED TO YOUR WEIGHT GAIN?

A. It is known that smokers weigh, on the average, a bit less than nonsmokers. The reasons for this are not entirely understood, but may be related to one or more of the following: the slight appetite-suppressing effect of cigarettes, altered taste preferences in smokers, or an altered metabolism due to nicotine. It is also common for smokers to gain weight when they quit smoking. The causes of this, too, are unclear, but include reversal of the previously mentioned effects of smoking as well as a tendency to use food, especially mood-elevating foods such as sweets and chocolate, as a substitute for cigarettes after quitting.

For the typical smoker, quitting is accompanied by a gain of about 6 pounds, but the amount is highly variable. One patient of mine reported gaining 80 pounds in the two years after he quit smoking.

Many people, in fact, choose not to quit smoking for fear that they will gain weight. Others go on a diet at the same time as attempting to quit in the hope of preventing weight gain. My research suggests that dieting is associated with greater levels of smoking in heavy smokers. Thus, dieting at the same time may make it even harder to quit smoking. Since smoking is generally more dangerous than weighing a bit more, it is unwise to resume smoking in an effort to control weight.

If you are someone who has gained more weight than average after quitting smoking, there is good news. There are specific strategies you can follow, and they do not include taking up smoking again. These strategies are described in detail on pages 92–93. They include increasing physical activity, eating fat-free sweets, chewing sugarless chewing gum, and drinking liquids after meals.

B. Just as the amount of weight gained during pregnancy is highly variable, so is the amount retained *after* pregnancy. Two years after pregnancy, the average woman weighs about 9 pounds more than she did prior to conception. This occurs with each pregnancy, of course. For women who have had several children or who had higher than average weight gain during a pregnancy, the numbers can add up to quite a few pounds. The causes are not well understood, but may include hormonal influences (women who do not breast-feed, for example, may be more likely to gain than those who do) and changes in lifestyle after having a baby (including less regular exercise).

There are specific things you can do to lose weight now, and to help prevent weight gain after future pregnancies. They include breast-feeding and getting down to or near prepregnancy weight before becoming pregnant again. The role of physical activity is critical, as is understanding other baby-associated lifestyle changes.

C. If you believe that a recent decrease in your physical activity is a major factor in causing you to gain weight, take heart. This specific cause is not only treatable, but the treatment yields benefits beyond helping you to lose weight. Chapter 7 tells you how to design an exercise plan that will fit your specific circumstances and will form an important part of your Personal Plan of Action.

The benefits of designing and carrying out a lifelong plan to increase physical activity include accelerating the pace of weight loss, making it much less likely that you will regain the weight you lose, and improving your cardiovascular fitness, stamina, and sense of well-being. As described further in Chapter 7, if you include a strength-training component in your Personal Plan, you will also build metabolically active muscle mass. This will enable you to eat a bit more than those who do only aerobic exercise and still not regain lost weight down the road.

D. Depression can contribute to either weight gain or weight loss. People who are feeling chronically down may have trouble motivating themselves for any kind of change or activity, including weight loss. The interaction between mood and eating is complex; I discuss it in more detail in Chapter 5. Here, it is important to distinguish between three categories of what people loosely call "depression."

The first is temporary, situational depression. This kind of depression occurs when something sad happens to you, like a death in the family. The second is unhappiness that stems from anxiety about or dissatisfaction with a specific part of your life (a relationship, a job, your appearance). The sadness that has a life of its own—that is not triggered by a specific life event or by unhappiness over some part of our life—is the third and generally the most serious form of depression. This kind of depression is considered to be a clinical illness, requiring medical treatment.

I find that most people who wish to lose weight and say that they are "depressed" fall into the second category, though many of them are clinically depressed. A few have suffered losses (category 1) and have gained weight because they eat to console themselves when sad.

The first and second types of depression are almost always temporary. Time heals almost all wounds. The use of food in times of unhappiness is not helpful, though. It does little to relieve the unhappiness, and it contributes to weight gain, which can lead to still more unhappiness and dissatisfaction. This inappropriate and ineffective use of food can be stopped. So if you find that you use food to console yourself, and that this has caused weight gain, you can incorporate the material on changing habits discussed on pages 77–79 of chapter 5 into your Personal Plan, and reap the benefits. You will attack the things that make you unhappy with weapons that work. Food is not the cure for unhappiness.

If you think you may fall into the third category, clinical depression, there is hope. Specific medications and psychotherapy are widely available and usually effective in controlling this form of depression. You should suspect that you might suffer from clinical depression if, in addition to feeling sad a lot, you have trouble sleeping and your sadness is not related to specific events but exists even when things seem to be going well. You should see a qualified psychologist or psychiatrist for help. A detailed questionnaire for depression is included in Chapter 5.

E. If weight gain has occurred after beginning a new medication, in many cases your physician will be able to substitute another that is less likely to affect your appetite. Indeed, some medications can be stopped entirely, particularly when the medications are prescribed for a condition that often improves with weight loss, such as hypertension or diabetes. Medications that commonly contribute to weight gain include: steroids and progestins, including oral contraceptives; oral antidiabetic agents; tricyclic antidepressants; phenothiazines (antipsychotics); and lithium for manic depression.

F. Even if none of the listed specific factors applies in your case, you may be able to identify others that do. Identifying specific causes of weight gain is a useful exercise, because the causes often suggest their own solutions.

If you can't think of any reasons for your weight gain, don't despair. You can still develop a Personal Plan that addresses your needs, but, as described in chapters 4 and 5, you may benefit from a period of *self-observation*. This often makes the difference between just another diet that fails in the long run, and making a permanent and satisfying change in your life.

3. ARE YOU UNDERGOING A LOT OF LIFE CHANGES OR STRESSES AT THIS TIME?

If you didn't check off any of the items listed, this is the ideal time to begin the preparation and action stages of a diet. The fewer the stresses and distractions, the easier it is to focus on the task of designing and carrying out your Personal Plan.

If you have checked off one or more recent, current, or imminent major life changes, you should assess how likely they are to interfere with your weight loss plans. For example, a recent serious illness from which you recovered two months ago may have no impact, or even a positive impact, on your desire and ability to make favorable lifestyle changes. On the other hand, a current illness is likely to seriously interfere with your ability to concentrate on your plan, and will probably interfere with the exercise portion of your plan.

Be completely honest with yourself regarding the likelihood of your stresses interfering with your Personal Plan. It is probably better to work on alleviating the stresses in your life before you begin your plan in earnest.

4. WHAT ARE THE MAJOR REASONS YOU WISH TO LOSE WEIGHT?

____ **To improve my appearance.** This is the most common reason given. While appearance can be a strong motivator, it is best to have other motivators as well. This is because losing to improve appearance is basically losing for others rather than for yourself. If your self-image is tied directly to your weight, this is a prescription for unhappiness and disappointment. While we do live in a society that values thinness, it is in many ways an arbitrary value, one that has been made in favor of stoutness rather than thinness in many other cultures and even in our own a couple of generations ago. Thus, whether you are thin or heavy is not a reflection on your character, but merely on the prejudice of our society. Allowing yourself to subscribe without question to the belief that thin is better is not only wrong, it devalues you as a person. Instead, it is healthier to understand and accept that our society is arbitrary and unfair in some of the characteristics it values. You may choose to be responsive to the cultural pressure to be thinner, but failure to do so does not make you any less valuable a person. Please remember this and believe it. It will help you if you decide to lose weight and don't succeed, but it will also help you to lose weight successfully.

____ **To improve health and reduce health risks.** This is certainly an important reason for wishing to lose weight. Unfortunately, it tends not to be very motivating for many people because you usually can't see any immediate health benefits. For example, someone who is advised by his or her doctor to lose weight after suffering a lifethreatening heart attack is likely to be highly motivated. This same person would not have been nearly as motivated if he or she had been given the same advice six months earlier. Most of us have a remarkable ability to believe that we are somehow exempt from health risks. Moreover, theoretical risks lack immediacy. These are worries for the future, and, after all, no one can predict the future with certainty.

If you are someone who has medical problems (hypertension, high cholesterol, diabetes, arthritis, etc.) that can be alleviated by weight loss, or if you are someone at increased risk of these problems because of your weight, you should be aware of this concept of immediacy. You may want to lose weight for health reasons but not be very motivated by the prospects of bad or worsening health. Or you may start out motivated but lose your resolve quickly.

To address this particular readiness problem, use the following two tools. They serve to keep the medical and personal consequences immediately accessible to you as you begin your Personal Plan.

First, *make a list*. This should include medical as well as personal benefits of losing weight. Keep your list in a convenient place (in the kitchen is helpful for some). Look at it each day.

Second, *use self-talk*. This, too, must be personalized. It must have meaning for you. For example, a 55-year-old man I worked with kept in his wallet a note his daughter had written on a paper napkin and slipped to him during a family dinner. It read, "Dad, I want you around for a long, long time. Please stop eating so much." He had suffered a heart attack three years previously, was seriously overweight, and had repeatedly been advised to lose weight by his physician. Previous half-hearted attempts to adhere to a diet had failed, however. The consequences of failing health were insufficient to drive him toward definitive action until he realized, through his daughter's written message, that there was much to live for. This shifted the balance sheet for him and helped him to stay the course when the barriers to successful change seemed insurmountable. He told me that he would take his daughter's message out of his wallet and read it whenever he felt his Personal Plan was not working. To create your own message regarding a long and healthful life, think about and write down all the benefits of weight loss. Talk to yourself about them often. This will give you an advantage in the process of successful change. (See pages 60–61 for a sampling of positive self-statements you might use.)

____ **To improve my energy level and fitness.** Much of what was discussed above under health reasons to lose weight also applies to this category. Improving energy level and fitness can be a strong motivator, but one that is not easily sustained. Focusing on a *specific benefit* to be obtained tends to be much more motivating than something general like "I don't want to feel tired all the time." For example, one young man I helped treat came up with two specific reasons for losing weight which proved to be very effective motivators for him. He said, "I have a one-and-a-half-year-old son who's now walking. I want to be able to get down on the ground and play with him." He felt very much left out of his son's life because of his weight. Second, his hobby had been repairing and renovating old automobiles, but he had given this up when he gained weight. He revealed, "I want to be able to fit under the cars to work on them." His abdomen had grown to the point where he was getting stuck on the way out.

Do you have specific things you used to do but are now unable to because of increased weight and decreased fitness? Examples include sports, hobbies, forms of transportation (riding the bus, bicycling, and fast walking) and specific activities (playing with children or grandchildren, running for airplanes without risking collapse). Use these specifics instead of generalities and you will find yourself more ready to change.

___ **To avoid the embarrassment of being overweight.** This reason is complex. It is similar to the already-discussed, "To improve my appearance." Because of our cultural peculiarities, it takes a high level of self-esteem or other defenses not to feel embarrassed by a weight problem. Although shame is a powerful motivator, it is important that the source of the shame be specifically identified and examined.

Stating this reason for losing weight in more positive terms is a better way to motivate yourself for the long term. A more positive statement is: "I want to feel good about my energy level, fitness, and comfort in socializing." Use specifics that apply to you when defining the benefits of weight loss.

___ **To please someone important to me.** This reason is discussed in detail below in regard to question number 5. *Beware of this reason.* You will improve your readiness for permanent change if you can find other reasons for losing weight than pleasing others.

You may have motivations for weight loss not discussed here. The important thing is that you carefully examine them and see whether they increase your readiness to begin and sustain an effective Personal Plan. Many do not.

For example, it is common for people to decide to lose weight because of an upcoming event like a wedding. This reason possesses many of the attributes that enhance readiness and motivation (it is important to you, very specific, and has immediacy). What it lacks, however, is long-term sustainability. What is likely to happen? Because of the pressure to lose weight by the wedding date the caloric deprivation required will be extreme, perhaps with an intensive exercise regimen as well. There is unlikely to be an emphasis on changing eating habits. Once the goal is achieved, or the wedding date arrives, the reason for losing weight departs with the guests, and old habits re-emerge with a vengeance. Clearly, this is not a good way to enhance long-term readiness.

In summary, you should evaluate your reasons for wanting to lose weight in terms of the following criteria:

Are they specific?
Are they important to you?
Do they have immediacy?
Do they meet your needs and not just the needs of others?
Can they sustain your motivation over the long term?

Each reason need not satisfy all five criteria, but the reasons *in total* should. Also, as pointed out above, you can reframe almost any reason to meet more of the five criteria through positive self-talk.

5. WHOM DO YOU WANT TO LOSE WEIGHT FOR?

In this era of self-help, most people know that the "correct" answer to the above question is to rank "myself" as the number one person. Why is this desirable? Because losing weight for you means that you have explored and have come to understand the personal benefits of losing weight, *for you*. It's easier in the long run to lose weight when you do it because losing weight makes *you* feel so much better physically than because it makes your spouse feel so proud of himself or herself for having a svelte partner. When your primary motivation is to please others, as in this example, there is a high likelihood that the motivation will not sustain you in the long run, and may even foster feelings of resentment toward the person you are trying to please.

Wishing to please a spouse or significant other is a very common reason for wanting to lose weight. For example, Sandy, a 30-year-old elementary school teacher, came to us for this reason. She had other reasons for wanting to lose weight, but her husband's disapproval was the strongest immediate motivator. It hurt her that her husband, Jack, said that he found her less desirable because of the weight she had gained (about 30 pounds) over the prior two years. The truth is that there were other problems in the relationship, as well. Interestingly, Sandy, like other people in her position, stated initially that she wished to lose weight primarily for herself, not for others. But this was simply not the case. Unfortunately, Sandy was not able to reframe her reasons more positively. She tried to lose weight but was unable to stick to her diet and exercise plan. She dropped out of the program within a month.

While other factors played a role in her lack of success, Sandy's lack of success stemmed from larger problems—an unhappy marriage, for one. The lesson to be learned here is that Sandy, like most people, was not likely to succeed in losing weight if she was doing it to please her spouse. The message her husband was sending her was a destructive one—in effect, he was saying, "My attraction and love for you is based on superficial rather than innate qualities you possess." Sandy might have done better if her marital problems had been addressed first, or if they had been addressed along with her weight problems.

Thus, it is important once again to examine your own motivations. Are you *really* doing this for you? You are much better off emphasizing the personal benefits you will reap through weight loss than being a martyr and doing it for someone else. You will greatly enhance your readiness for permanent change if you are able to convince yourself that this is so. You are going to develop a Personal Plan for you, because *you* want to change.

6. HOW MUCH WEIGHT DO YOU WISH TO LOSE?

There is no right answer here, so let's look at the choices, and how your choice can impact both your readiness and the likelihood of achieving short- and long-term success.

A. Goal: ideal body weight or less. Ideal body weight is a standard based on weights of young, middle-class Caucasian men and women. Aiming for ideal body weight may be reasonable in some cases but not in others. If you have always been in this range as an adult but gained weight after a specific event like a pregnancy or quitting smoking, it is certainly possible for you to get back to your normal weight. It is never a good idea to aim for a weight lower than ideal body weight. Not only are you unlikely to sustain such a weight, it may be unhealthy for you to do so.

For most of the people who need to lose weight, however, ideal body weight is not a wise goal. If you have never been in this range, or last saw it on your sixteenth birthday, it is a virtual certainty that you will not be able to achieve or sustain that goal weight. Nor do you need to. As discussed, health risks seem to be minimal with modest degrees of overweight. Aiming for "ideal" body weight is usually aiming for frustration. Not recommended.

B. Goal: most of the way to ideal body weight. This goal may be a reasonable one, but that will depend on a realistic assessment of your personal weight history. Again, if you have never been anywhere near "ideal" body weight, an initial goal even two-thirds of the way there may be unreasonable. For instance, if your ideal body weight is 125–135 pounds but your usual weight has been 220 pounds, you would be aiming for a weight of 160 pounds, a loss of 60 pounds, more than a quarter of your total starting body weight. While this is by no means impossible, it is a major task to attain and maintain such a goal weight.

On the other hand, if your ideal body weight is also 125–135 pounds but your current weight is only 160 pounds, and you've been in the 140-pound range in the past, it is quite reasonable to set a goal of ⅔ of the way to ideal body weight. This would entail a loss of 20 pounds, to 140 pounds.

C. Goal: enough to feel more comfortable and reduce health risks. This is a common goal for people who have been very overweight for most of their lives. It is the most attainable and sustainable kind of goal. In many cases it is not necessary to put an exact number on it, since you may not know what weight improves physical comfort and health until you reach it. For many people who are seriously overweight, a loss of even 10 percent of their body weight, for example 20 pounds for a 200-pound woman, is likely to improve health risks, like high blood pressure, and fitness level. While such a goal may not put you near our cultural "ideals" for weight, it can have a very major impact on the quality of your life. Such a goal should not be disparaged, only admired.

There is a tendency to believe that setting goals that are very difficult to achieve improves the ultimate outcome—this is called "reach for the stars" reasoning. While striving for the nearly impossible is part of our folklore, and much admired, it works well only for the rare individual blessed with skill, drive, and luck. In weight loss, reaching for the stars is almost certain to result in disappointment, and reflects a lack of appreciation for the magnitude of the task. Unreasonable goals will make even successful weight loss seem like a failure. In other words, if you cannot set goals that are reasonable for your personal situation, you are not ready to begin your Personal Plan.

What, then, is a reasonable goal weight for you? With the above discussion and the material in chapters 4 and 6, you can set an appropriate goal and have the best chance of attaining and sustaining it.

7. HOW MUCH HAVE YOU DIETED IN THE PAST?

A. Never. This is often a good thing. You will not have had the experience of losing weight, then gaining it back. You probably have fewer preconceived notions about dieting and the likely outcome of your diet efforts. In general, we find that first-time dieters at the Johns Hopkins Weight Management Center have a very good chance of successfully completing their diet.

B. I've dieted one to a few times before. This means that you have some previous experience with attempting to lose weight but are not a frequent dieter. In an age where a majority of adults have dieted at least once, you are clearly not alone. Most people diet on their own, sometimes with the help of friends or books like this one, rather than through a formal program. Read the discussion of choice C to see what can be learned from your previous diet attempts.

C. I've dieted four or more times before. Although this sounds like a lot of times, it may reassure you to know that you are not alone. In any given year in the United States, 45 to 47 percent of women and 25 to 30 percent of men have dieted. Even if you have been initially successful in your previous diet attempts, having to repeat these efforts can be discouraging.

To enhance your readiness for long-lasting changes this time, you must view the previous dieting as valuable experience for the successful plan you are about to begin. In fact, previous diets do offer lessons you can learn from. In this way, then, you have an advantage over people who have never dieted before. I urge you to use this advantage to the fullest.

For example, you may, in retrospect, have wanted to do things differently during or after a diet. Perhaps you began a previous diet when you were unable to commit the needed time and energy to the process, and now can. Perhaps you were dieting for the wrong reasons on a previous diet, and know better now. Perhaps you were doing it for someone else in the past, and will do it for you this time. Perhaps you had no coherent strategy during and after a previous diet, but this time you will formulate a Personal Plan of Action to see you through. Fill in the blanks below. Think about your answers and write them down.

In the past I _____ ,

but this time I will _____ .

Also in the past I _____ ,

but this time I will _____ .

Now you can see how to make previous diets help your current effort. This is a very practical use of your valuable past experience, and will greatly enhance your readiness to change. I advise you to take full advantage of your personal dieting history—then you are much less likely to relive it.

8. WHAT WAS THE TYPICAL SHORT-TERM OUTCOME OF PREVIOUS DIETS?

A. I reached my goal weight. Congratulations! You clearly have sufficient motivation to lose weight during the action phase. Since you have done it before, I'd venture to say that you can do it again. This time, you will be following a plan that *you* will devise to meet your specific needs. You will be applying your considerable tenacity not just to a diet, but to a comprehensive Personal Plan that addresses the habits causing you to gain or regain weight. This should be no more difficult for you than sticking with a traditional diet, because you will have less deprivation on your Personal Plan. The emphasis will be on dieting smart, making shrewd substitutions for the foods that get you into trouble, and recognizing and changing inappropriate eating habits. The emphasis will not be on using sheer willpower to stick to a very restrictive diet plan. The fact that you have the proven ability to reach your short-term goals even on a "brute-force" diet should make you feel quite confident about your ability to succeed with your own Personal Plan of Action.

B. I got at least halfway to my goal. Congratulations again! Considering that most people seem to set their goals too aggressively, getting at least halfway there is usually quite an accomplishment. Too often, we focus on the part not achieved, rather than the considerable amount that was achieved. This is obviously self-defeating. It will be best if you do not fall into this trap as you prepare your Personal Plan. You will be setting reasonable goals, with a plan geared to your specific needs, with a minimum of deprivation. That you were able in the past to get at least halfway to your goal without a Personal Plan is good evidence that you can do even better *with* one.

C. I got less than halfway to my goal. Discouraging, isn't it? You don't believe you can do much better this time. Well, maybe you are wrong. Try looking at it this way. You can learn quite a lot from past experience. Read the discussion of answer 7C above, and fill in the blanks if you have not already done so. If you set reasonable goals, develop well-thought-out reasons for losing weight, carefully devise your own Personal Plan as described in chapters 4–7, and talk positively to yourself about your ability to change, you will do remarkably well, regardless of your previous history.

9. WHAT WAS THE TYPICAL OUTCOME OF PREVIOUS DIETS (LONG TERM)?

A. I kept off most of the weight for many years. You are to be congratulated. You are in a select minority. If you have now regained, it is likely that some specific factor is involved in your regain of weight. If you have not regained and are still quite heavy, you may wish to lose more weight. In either case it is likely that you will again prove successful in controlling your weight problem. Take advantage of the guidance available in these chapters, and begin with confidence.

B. I regained the weight after keeping most of it off for two or more years. This, too, is an accomplishment to be proud of. Considering how common yo-yo dieting is, maintaining a majority of the weight lost during a diet for two or more years afterwards is excellent. To do this, you had to succeed in continuing some form of diet and/or exercise-related behavior change for at least two years. It will be unhelpful if you focus on the fact that you eventually regained. Instead, take justifiable pride in the fact that you were able to sustain real behavior change for a prolonged period of time. If you could do that in the past, you can surely do it again now. And now you will have the advantage of past experience, and an individualized program that will help you to address those specific areas that are causing problems for you now.

C. I regained the weight after keeping most of it off for less than two years. Although this can be discouraging, here too, there is valuable information to be gathered. Above all, don't get down on yourself for weight regain. View the past as objectively as you can. There can be many reasons why someone regains weight, and you can benefit from examining several different categories. These include your motivators for weight loss (see questions 4 and 5), the stresses and other circumstances that you lived through in the postdiet period (question 3), whether your weight goals were reasonable for you (question 6), whether you focused on changing your long-term eating habits or just taking off pounds, and any specific causes of weight gain that may have appeared in the postdiet period.

The bottom line is that you can learn more from mistakes than from success. Do it differently this time, and past mistakes become irrelevant. You will be better able to do it right this time, for keeps, if you learn from your past and incorporate this hard-earned wisdom into your Personal Plan.

10. HOW WILL YOU BEHAVE WHILE DIETING?

A. I will likely have a very hard time adhering to my plan. If you believe this to be true, there are at least two things to be aware of. First, your belief that things will not go well is undoubtedly arising from your past experience in attempting to lose weight. As you are now aware, a bad past experience can be quite useful—*you can learn from it*. Second, your belief that you will be unable to adhere to a weight loss plan has a tendency to make it harder to alter that dire prediction. It becomes a self-fulfilling prophecy—if you believe you will fail, you will fail. This is not the desired outcome, and such negative beliefs, no matter how compelling, based on past experience, must be countered. To counter them you can engage in positive self-talk and positive action.

Analyze why you believe you will experience difficulty. What did you do in the past that may have sabotaged your ability to stick with your plans? Was the diet you tried too limiting, entailing too much deprivation? Was the timing of the attempt wrong because of concurrent stresses? Were your goals unreasonable or not focused on behavior changes? Did you lack a good support system? Were you not convinced of the need to change at that time? All of your answers are important, because all these conditions can be changed this time to help you through. All that's required is a carefully thought out Personal Plan, and your positive beliefs and actions.

B. I will likely be spotty in adhering to my plan. Read the discussion in answer 10A, because it applies equally well to this situation. Basically, you should try to figure out what leads to your belief that your behavior will not be consistent. With what you have learned from past experience, you can set up your current goals, timing, motivators, support systems, and specific aspects of your diet and physical activity program so that you will be able to adhere consistently to your Personal Plan during the action phase.

C. I will likely be consistently compliant with my plan. Congratulations! You either have had good success in complying with past diets or have taken to heart the advice to think positively. There is only one potential down side to consistent compliance during the action phase of a weight loss plan. Some people have little trouble with the initial adherence to a regimen but are prone to "all-or-nothing" behavior. To oversimplify, they are either being really compliant with a strict diet or being really out of control of their eating, with no intermediate mode of behavior. If you think you are prone to "all-or-nothing" behavior, there are some things you can build into your Personal Plan that will help you to strike a healthy balance. These are discussed in Chapter 5, "Why Do You Eat?"

For the purpose of increasing readiness, anyone in Category C (or even Category B) should understand that the ability to adhere to a diet, even if only for a while, is very valuable. The results you will see when you adhere to your Personal Plan will be very gratifying. They will help you to continue your plan to completion and beyond.

11. HOW WILL YOU BEHAVE AFTER THE ACTIVE DIETING PHASE HAS BEEN COMPLETED?

A. I will likely go right back to old habits. Assuming that you are responding this way based on your past experience, one of the most important things you can do is examine your past behavior, so you can learn from it. Were you dieting just for a specific occasion like a family wedding? Were you not convinced of the need for long-lasting changes in your behavior? You can feel more confident this time, because before you begin you will have your ducks all lined up—you will have a Personal Plan of Action that includes ways to make the changes last.

B. I will likely start out with good habits then slowly revert to the old habits. This is a very common pattern. As discussed previously, readiness has a tendency to fade with time. To maintain behavior changes beyond the action stage, a new set of skills is needed. These include repetition, making your environment work for you, keeping track of your behavior, and using flexible responses. All of these tools can be learned, and are discussed in detail in Chapter 4 and again in Chapter 8. You will be incorporating many of them into your Personal Plan.

C. I will likely maintain the good new habits for a long time. Congratulations! That is the most important thing to be accomplished through your Personal Plan. Feeling confident that you will be able to maintain positive behavior changes indefinitely will help you to do so.

12. WHAT FACTORS WILL PLAY AN IMPORTANT ROLE IN PREVENTING YOU FROM SUCCESSFULLY COMPLETING A WEIGHT LOSS PLAN?

____ **Lack of time.** To increase your readiness for change, it is important that you be realistic about how much time and energy you are willing and able to commit to this endeavor. If you decide to proceed, you will be better prepared (more ready) if you make a specific time commitment on a regular, scheduled basis. For example, the typical client at the Johns Hopkins Weight Management Center is asked to schedule about one hour per day for meal planning and preparation, one-half hour per day for exercise, and one to two hours per week for "school"—attending a group class and seeing the physician, dietician, or psychologist. A similar schedule will apply to you and your Personal Plan. You will need time to plan meals so that you are not subject to the enticement of fast food, you will need to schedule a time for regular physical activity, and you will need time to do your "schoolwork" at home. Your schoolwork will consist of recording your activities and progress in your Personal Plan.

Many people believe that they won't have the time to follow a weight loss plan properly. This is not often the case. To increase your readiness, you should remind yourself how important losing weight is for you. Surely you spend some of your time in ways that are a lot less important to you. In fact, through a little creative time management, you can continue virtually all your previous activities and still devote enough time to your Personal Plan. Making other functions serve dual roles is the key to this technique of time management. For instance, exercising while watching TV is a great time saver, and has the added benefit of making it impossible to eat while watching TV. When you incorporate this kind of time saver into your Personal Plan, you need never again say, "I don't have the time." You do, and you must use it.

_____ **Lack of physical resources.** Lack of physical resources, namely, the funds to purchase exercise equipment, personal counseling, classes, and the like is not necessarily an impediment to weight loss. In fact, there is some evidence that people are often more successful in keeping weight off long-term on their own than through formal programs. Most formal weight loss programs treat everyone very much the same, and fail to take into account the crucial differences between Sally, Jane, and Tim, each of whom needs to lose the same 40 pounds. Formal programs sometimes do not provide support during the all-important maintenance stage. Thus, it is quite feasible for you, with no more physical resources than this guide and your own commitment and planning, to achieve the goals you set in your Personal Plan.

On the other hand, studies have shown that investing a significant amount of your physical resources in this endeavor to lose weight and keep it off can be a very potent motivator. When people are given financial incentives to adhere to a program (for example, refund of a substantial deposit), they tend to do better. People who are given services free of charge, conversely, often drop out of a program, and rarely do very well even if they stay. While there are many tales of expensive exercise equipment gathering dust in a corner, you can only get the benefits from such equipment if you own it. Having a financial and physical investment in your Personal Plan can make it more likely that you will follow through on it. The financial cost of devising and carrying out your Personal Plan can be nothing, or quite considerable. While it is sometimes helpful to have an "investment" in your plan, the lack of one does not mean you cannot carry out your plan successfully. Therefore, lack of physical or financial resources need not affect your readiness and commitment to change.

____ **Lack of motivation.** This is the most commonly cited impediment to change. But it is meaningless in and of itself. As we have discussed, lack of motivation usually reflects a lack of planning. In the past, you may have fallen victim to lack of motivation midway through a diet, perhaps when results were not as good as you had hoped, or the diet was more difficult than advertised, or the wedding was over.

This time can be different. You have already examined, and will continue to reevaluate, your good reasons for embarking on this course of action. You will devise a plan that takes into account your specific needs as an individual. You will have reasonable goals, a strong support system, and the flexibility to adjust your plan to changing circumstances. In short, lack of motivation is not an ingredient in your Personal Plan. You will be well prepared this time. You are ready.

____ **Lack of support from family or significant others.** This, too, can be very complex. Your best chance for success lies in having "pleasing yourself" as your primary reason for embarking on a weight loss plan. Bearing in mind the benefits you will obtain from successfully losing weight and keeping it off will help you to stay motivated. Sometimes, though, spouses or others, for reasons they may not even understand, will behave in an unsupportive or even a destructive manner. They may be jealous of your resolve or success. They may feel threatened. They may simply be unaware that their behavior is making it harder for you to adhere to your Personal Plan.

There is less of a chance that this problem will derail your plans this time around. Your motivations and coping skills will be stronger. You will probably build a "buddy system" of support into your Personal Plan. If you have decided to do this plan *for you,* pleasing others is not the point. While you cannot always control the behavior of others, you can control your own response to others' behavior. Because you will be aware of the unsupportive behavior of other people, you will be able to choose how to respond. You may decide that their behavior is irrelevant and choose to ignore it or to separate yourself physically from it. For example, you may choose to eat at a different time or in a different place when co-workers order in fast food for lunch and offer you some. Or, in the same situation, you may instead decide to address the unsupportive behavior directly. You can ask that your colleagues not make such offers because it makes it harder for you to adhere to your diet.

When the unsupportive person is a spouse or someone else who is very close to you, you may decide to explore what's behind this behavior. Perhaps the other person is unaware of the behavior or the effect it has on you. In this case, you'll need to tell the person what effect it has on you. You can strengthen your coping skills by letting him or her know exactly what you would like him or her to do to be supportive. You may need to do this repeatedly. Whether the unsupportive person responds positively or not, you can stay on track (see Chapter 5 for a more complete discussion of how to handle the would-be saboteur). You can rely on yourself and the Personal Plan you have devised for support.

If you have a supportive family member, you are in the best position to achieve your weight loss goals. Remember Aaron, the architect, whom we discussed earlier in this chapter? Even though Aaron's wife didn't appear on Aaron's balance sheet, she did all the cooking, and this was one reason Aaron had trouble losing weight. If Aaron's wife were actively included in his Personal Plan, however, Aaron's chances of success would be greatly improved. In fact, he and his wife could find that learning to cook together in new, healthier ways is a great hobby they both can share. Cooking, shopping, and even eating could become positive experiences, and the couple's time together could become one of the positive things about Aaron's losing weight.

While it can be helpful to get the unqualified support of others, always remember that, by far, your most important booster is you.

——**Major stressful events intrude.** Many people have a tendency to abandon "optional" activities like losing weight and fall back on tried-and-true coping mechanisms like eating when stressful events occur. These old habits are tried, but they are not usually true. That is, *they don't work*. Although major stresses are indeed disruptive, eating does nothing to help a person deal with them. With luck, a major stress will not intrude anytime during or shortly after the action stage of your Personal Plan. If one does, though, you will be prepared. Your plan will include ways to deal appropriately with stress, without resorting to excess eating. Knowing that you have learned other ways to deal with major (and minor) stresses can make you less fearful of this form of intrusion into your plans. You are ready.

___ **Need to lose weight becomes less important.** This is a near-universal phenomenon. It can occur at two different times. First, it can occur early in the action stage, before you have come close to your goal. Second, it can occur late in the action stage or during maintenance, when you have nearly reached your goal.

When it strikes early in the action stage, the cause is often lack of strong personal reasons for wanting to lose weight. This need not happen to you, because you have examined your reasons and understand how to formulate them so they emphasize the benefits to you in losing weight, so they are specific, so they have immediacy, and so they are important and can sustain your motivation. Your Personal Plan will include reminders of why you are committed to losing weight, which you can refer to when you think you are forgetting their importance.

When it strikes late, when you are near your goal or in maintenance, the cause is often a false sense of security. You have gotten through the worst of it, you may believe. You have already obtained most of the benefits of weight loss. The last bit seems less important. What we can say from experience is: Not really. This time you have a greater respect and appreciation for the difficulties of maintaining weight loss, and have incorporated maintenance into your Personal Plan from Day 1. You will not let down your guard when you near your goal, nor when you achieve it. You are ready for long-term success.

Now that you have analyzed your past experience and current thinking, you have completed the hardest part of the task of making the most of your state of readiness for change. What remains is to set out some rules, and to condition your environment so that it supports your goals.

First, the rules:

1. Remember: you are doing this for you, not for others.
2. Keep the benefits to you in the foreground—update your Personal Balance Sheet on a regular basis.
3. Make the goals reasonable.

4. Monitor your progress regularly.
5. Vow to analyze and learn from past and future mistakes.

Now, set the conditions that will help you get started:

1. Clear the decks: make time for formulating and carrying out your Personal Plan.
2. Make your home a safe place for carrying out your plan: clear the kitchen of temptations.
3. Find a dieting partner, if possible (see Chapter 4).
4. Pick a reasonable goal weight (Chapter 2) and specific behavior goals (Chapter 5), a diet (Chapter 6), and an exercise plan (Chapter 7).

As a final bit of encouragement, consider this. You do difficult things every day. The boss gives you a terribly unpleasant task to do. There is no one else who can do it, and so you do it. At home, at work, at school, in the community—there are a zillion difficult things to be done, and you do them. The trick with weight loss and maintenance is to convince yourself, with the help of the tools described in this chapter, that this course of action is not a matter of preference, but of necessity. It's not that you should lose weight someday. You have decided that you will, that you must, that it is your duty to yourself, a duty you can no more shirk than comforting your frightened child crying out in the dead of night. You are already well on your way to the action stage, so let's get going.

THREE

Beginning Your Self-Assessment

Imagine the setting: a medium-sized conference room on the first floor of an office building. Around a conference table on this wintery Tuesday evening sit twelve people, ten women and two men, who have gathered after work for a meeting. This is a diverse group brought together by one thing—they are all obese, and they all are very serious about wanting to lose weight. The purpose of the meeting is to hear about the approach offered by the staff of the Johns Hopkins Weight Management Center to help people lose weight and keep it off. Most of the people in this orientation meeting have dieted before, some many times, but none successfully in the long run.

The members of the group range in age from 20 to 68. They come from all walks of life—from college student to executive; from secretary to restaurant owner. They are equally different in income, race, and religion. The factors that led to their current weight problem are also quite varied. A few have been heavy since childhood, but most did not become overweight until their late teens or adult life. Some have horrendous eating habits, living almost exclusively on junk food, while others claim to eat a nutritious, varied diet full of fresh fruits, vegetables, and grains. Most are physically inactive, but one plays tennis regularly and another runs religiously three times each week.

The most interesting thing about this group is that their diversity is typical of people who want to lose weight. The 60-year-old restaurant owner who loves rich foods is clearly very different from the 35-year-old who has recently undergone a difficult divorce and gained weight in the process—even though they are both women and are both 55 pounds over their "ideal" weight. But even if you selected twelve equally overweight women of the same age and occupation and race, and from the same town, you would be likely to find that each one of them is overweight for a different set of reasons.

Our approach to weight loss recognizes these individual differences and uses them to formulate the best diet plan for each person. Why is this individualization so important? Won't everyone lose weight if they just follow a strict diet? Who cares how the person became heavy in the first place?

The fact is that, yes, everyone loses weight when they cut their intake of calories below their energy usage. Unfortunately, as many people have experienced firsthand, the diet won't last forever, and when the diet ends, weight tends to be regained, sometimes with distressing rapidity. One thing that leads to regaining weight after a diet is that most diets don't address the *habits* that contributed to unwanted weight gain. The diet is often a short-term success but a long-term failure, because it has provided little or no guidance about how to behave after the diet phase has ended. This kind of guidance is crucial to long-term weight loss. To be effective, a diet must be *individualized* to address the areas that cause problems for each individual person.

For example, it would make little sense to teach the 60-year-old-restaurateur how to avoid eating to relieve emotional distress; this is not one of her problem areas. Similarly, the 35-year-old divorcee already knows a lot about good nutrition and practices it—unless she is under emotional stress. Moreover, neither of them will be helped to conquer her weight problem in the long term by simply being placed on the typical low-calorie diet. They will both lose some weight, but only temporarily.

We believe that individualization is simply common sense: what works best is a low-calorie diet *combined with* an individualized blueprint for change. Our focus is on altering the habits that caused the weight problem in the first place. The tool for accomplishing this individualization is a personalized assessment of each person's state of readiness, as well as his or her medical, dietary, behavioral, and exercise profiles. These assessments provide information that helps us plan the solutions that will work best for each individual. The blueprint which results from this planning process is what we call a Personal Plan. It is a plan of action, a plan designed by working from the specific needs of the individual.

The assessment process is critical to the development of a Personal Plan of Action. At the Johns Hopkins Weight Management Center, the assessment is done by a team of experts in the disciplines most relevant to the weight management process, and the various assessments add up to a *comprehensive assessment*. The team consists of:

a *physician,* to assess the person's medical status and develop a medical risk profile;

a *dietician,* to assess the person's current diet and offer suggestions for change;

a *psychologist,* to assess personal habits (the "why" of eating) and enhance personal readiness for change;

and an *exercise physiologist,* to assess the person's current level of physical fitness, and suggest improvements and variations to burn up more calories.

The different parts of the assessment overlap and interact with each other in various ways that can improve progress in weight loss.

Obviously, not everyone has access to such a team of experts. Except for the medical evaluation, most people will be able to conduct a detailed self-assessment using this book alone. However, some people will need professional help with some parts of the assessment; the information contained in this book will help you determine if *you* do. After the assessment, I will explain how you can use the information gained to formulate your own Personal Plan of Action.

First, a word about commitment, or what some people call the "buy in." A crucial factor in your decision to adopt the Weight Management Center's approach to weight loss is whether you agree that a good deal of effort will be required if you commit yourself to the program. If you believe that this work of self-understanding and behavior change is essential for long-term success, then read on. You have probably done a certain amount of soul-searching in order to get this far. More will surely follow if you make the decision to proceed.

Now, if you have completed the questionnaire in the previous chapter and have thought about ways to enhance your readiness to change, you already know about developing a Personal Plan. You understand the importance of making gradual lifestyle changes, and of acquiring the tools to make your changes a permanent part of your life. You are well beyond the contemplation stage and are actively preparing for change. Let's proceed to the rest of the assessment process—the medical, dietary, behavioral, and physical activity assessments. The order in which the assessments are done doesn't matter, but the individualized plan is not complete without the final synthesis, when input from each of the assessments is combined to form a comprehensive picture of you and the steps you will take to ensure your success in the action stage—and beyond.

The Medical Assessment

Unlike the other assessments, the medical assessment *must* be performed by a trained professional, a physician. In addition to assessing your overall health, the physician will concentrate on four areas while evaluating you before you begin a weight loss program. First, the physician will assess the medical consequences that being overweight has imposed, or is at risk of imposing, on your health. Second, she or he will determine whether your current medical treatment, if any, is in conflict with the weight loss plan you are about to undertake. Third, the physician will discuss the pros and cons of various weight loss techniques—rapid versus slower, diet versus exercise, and others. Fourth, the two of you will talk about your hopes, fears, and aspirations; a good internist or family practitioner will be able to address these issues in a forthright but empathetic way. (You may need to interview several physicians to find someone who can best meet your needs.)

Generally speaking, there are three parts to a medical assessment: (1) the medical history, (2) the physical examination, and (3) laboratory testing (when necessary). The physical examination and necessary laboratory testing can be done only by a physician. The physician will also take your medical history. In fact, since a carefully taken medical history is often far more revealing than the physical examination, most physicians start there. I begin the medical assessment of my weight loss patients with a medical history, focusing on the clues revealed by the history to help them develop a Personal Plan. Most doctors use a standardized format when taking a patient's history, generally following this order:

Chief Complaint	(CC)
History of Present Illness	(HPI)
Past History	(PH)
Family History	(FH)
Social History	(SH)
Review of Systems	(ROS)

As an exercise, let's imagine you are seeing me for a medical assessment. I am going to ask you some questions. Unfortunately, I can't hear your responses, so you will have to write them down. I can't see them, either, so you will have to interpret the answers as best you can with some general guidance from me. You must also understand that *this is only an exercise,* and you must not act or fail to act based on this exercise. Before beginning a diet, consult your physician in person for a medical history and physical, especially if you suspect or know that you have medical problems, if you are age 60 or older or 17 or younger, or if you are pregnant or breastfeeding. Now let's begin the medical history exercise.

Chief Complaint. In my early days of training to become a doctor I learned that it's not a good idea to ask a patient about the chief complaint by saying, "So, what brings you here today?" One portly older gentlemen replied, deadpan, "my wife." I wasn't sure, then, whether he was misinterpreting the question (his wife drove the car) or revealing a profound truth (his wife forced him to see me). In the light of my 20 years of subsequent training and experience, though, I now believe he was simply laughing at me.

How about *your* chief complaint? The chief complaint is traditionally recorded in the medical record in the patient's own words, in quotes, like this:

CC: "I'm so fat I have trouble . . ."

You need to be specific, since, as you recall from Chapter 2, the more specific and personal and positive your goals are, the better your results will be. Write your chief reason for wanting to lose weight here:

CC: "＿＿＿＿＿＿＿＿＿＿＿＿＿＿＿＿＿＿＿＿＿＿＿＿"

What can you learn from your answer? The discussion of the various answers to question 4 in Chapter 2 will provide some insight.

History of Present Illness. The HPI is elicited by asking the patient such open-ended questions as, "When did you first notice the problem?" "What symptoms or consequences did it have?" "What happened next?" and "What do you think is contributing to the problem?"

The significance of your answers may be understood, at least in part, by reading the discussions of questions 1, 2, and 3 in Chapter 2. For the purpose of this medical self-assessment, I would like you to focus on the physical limitations your weight problem may have caused, and the health, fitness, and quality-of-life improvements you stand to enjoy by losing weight. The "Review of Systems" section in this chapter will help you identify the symptoms you might be asking yourself about.

Past History refers to medical, surgical, or psychiatric problems other than those described under the HPI. It includes medications, hospitalizations, and other care, from birth to the present. These past and present problems may be relevant to the chief complaint; in addition, they serve as a reminder that the chief complaint has consequences beyond the obvious. For example, as discussed in Chapter 1, heart disease, high blood pressure, diabetes, arthritis, gout, low back pain, and various other ailments are often the result of, or are made worse by, a weight problem. If you have had any of these conditions or have symptoms of them, you should be under the care of a physician (see "Review of Systems," below). Because you have medical problems or have had them in the past usually does not mean that you should not lose weight. On the contrary, it may give you another good reason to lose.

Family History is important because genetics plays a significant role in determining whether you are likely to become overweight, and also whether you will suffer from various illnesses. The most common illnesses and conditions with a strong inherited component include heart disease, diabetes, certain cancers, high blood pressure, and high cholesterol and triglycerides.

How many of your close relatives (parents, grandparents, brothers, and sisters) are or were obese? Do any suffer from inherited illnesses or from conditions (heart disease, diabetes, stroke, arthritis, gout, high blood pressure, low back pain, high cholesterol or triglycerides) that obesity can cause or make worse? If any close relative is obese or suffers from these conditions, you may be at increased risk yourself. Losing weight now can reduce your risk and increase your fitness as well.

Social History refers to your living arrangements, job, education, and various medically relevant habits such as whether you smoke and how much alcohol you consume. All of these things can have an impact on your weight and how you should approach weight loss. (See the discussion of questions 2, 3, and 12 in Chapter 2.)

For example, if you are living alone, you may have an easier time making your home a temptation-free zone than if you are living with a spouse and children who seem to require vast quantities of food to sustain them. A stressful job may have led you to use food to cope. Your previous education may or may not have taught you about the principles of good nutrition. Bearing children and quitting smoking can lead to weight gains. Drinking a significant amount of alcohol is important both as a potential addiction and because it contributes a lot of "empty" calories (see Chapter 6).

Write down any of the features of your social history that will influence how you design your Personal Plan. It's important to remember to incorporate into your plan some way of dealing with these circumstances.

Review of Systems is a systematic series of questions designed to uncover possible health problems that you may not be aware of. The following is an abbreviated version of the standard ROS; this version emphasizes causes of, or problems that result from, being overweight.

REVIEW OF SYSTEMS

Do you suffer from any of these symptoms or illnesses, or have you suffered from them in the past?

General

Excessive fatigue? ___

Sleep disturbance? ___

Change in appetite? ___

Unexplained fever or chills? ___

Endocrine

Heat or cold intolerance? ___

Excessive thirst or urination? ___

Change in sex drive? ___

Excess hair growth? ___

Abnormal or absent periods? ___

Cardiopulmonary

High blood pressure? ___

Rheumatic heart disease or scarlet fever? ___

Inherited heart condition? ___

Chest pains? ___

Shortness of breath

with modest exertion? ___

when lying flat? ___

Wheezing? ___ Chronic cough? ___

Leg pain while walking? ___

Ankle swelling? ___

Gastrointestinal

Frequent heartburn? ___

Change in bowel habits? ___

Bleeding? ___

Abdominal pains? ___

Nausea/vomiting? ___

Neurologic/psychological

Dizziness? ___

Numbness/tingling? ___

Blackouts? ___

Weakness? ___

Seizures? ___

Anxiety? ___

Depression? ___

Suicide thoughts/attempts? ___

If you experience any of the symptoms listed in the ROS, consult your physician. It is unlikely that having any of these symptoms will mean that you cannot or should not lose weight. Rather, they may provide additional motivation for weight loss.

In some cases, the symptom can lead to a diagnosis that makes it easier to lose weight. This was the case for Anna, a 37-year-old executive assistant who reported fatigue and cold intolerance on her ROS. Upon further evaluation, we learned that she was suffering from hypothyroidism (underactivity of the thyroid gland, which produces hormones that regulate our metabolism). Treatment of her hypothyroidism made it much easier for Anna to lose weight.

In people like Anna, weight loss is easier or occurs automatically once their disease is treated. It is best not to expect this, however. Fewer than one in a hundred people with a weight problem have gained weight because of an endocrine disorder.

A much more likely result of seeing a physician about any symptoms you checked off on your ROS is that you will learn that you have a specific medical problem. Many medical problems can be treated or even "cured" by losing weight and keeping it off. For example, Jim, a 56-year-old engineer, reported that he was getting progressively more short of breath with physical exertion. This turned out to be a result of an early case of congestive heart failure with high blood pressure. In Jim's case, treatment of his high blood pressure and congestive heart failure with medications did not result in weight loss, because these problems were not a cause of his weight gain in the first place. The medications did, however, improve his shortness of breath and blood pressure. Even better, though, was Jim's motivation once he discovered these medical conditions. He lost almost 50 pounds over a period of 6 months through a Personal Plan which was geared to his specific problem areas, and he has kept the weight off.

Jim's motivation to maintain his new, lower weight has been boosted by the fact that weight loss made it possible for him to control his high blood pressure and mild heart condition *without* medications. The weight loss in combination with a low-salt diet enabled him to stop the medicines only a few months after they had been started.

Finally, Miriam, a very overweight 40-year-old sales associate, reported during her medical history that she often ate to settle her stomach. For the past four years she had been experiencing abdominal pains in between meals and in the late evening. She had not seen a physician. It turned out that she had chronic ulcers, which were easily treated with a three-week course of anti-ulcer medications. Eating to relieve her ulcer symptoms had not cured her ulcer. It had, however, caused her to gain 70 pounds in four years. The information that she had ulcers was very helpful to Miriam, who was able to keep her weight under control once she lost it with her Personal Plan. She no longer had the pain from her ulcers, so she didn't need to eat to try to feel better.

As noted earlier, the medical history is followed by a physical exam and laboratory tests, if needed, to complete the medical assessment. A careful medical assessment can provide a great deal of useful information about your health, and your health risks. If you do have a problem, it will often be one that is related to your weight in some way. Even if the problem is not one that tends to improve with weight loss, you will almost always benefit from finding out about the problem and getting expert medical treatment.

The Dietary Assessment

In our weight loss center, dietary assessments are performed by a registered dietician. I recommend that you consult a professional dietician, as well, if possible. But with the information in this book, you can conduct a very informative dietary self-assessment. The aims of this assessment are as follows:

1. To define your current weight category and weight history.
2. To determine your usual diet, including the percentage of your

intake from fats, your food preferences, and your meal
pattern.

3. To determine your body fat distribution pattern.
4. To develop an individualized weight-reducing diet.
5. To develop an individualized weight maintenance diet.

Because the dietary assessment is so important, a highly detailed
self-assessment is included in Chapter 6, "What's a 'Good' Diet, Anyway?" To develop your Personal Plan, it's essential that you complete
the exercises in Chapter 6.

For our purposes here, though, please consider the following points
right now. The dietary assessment will be useful to you only if you are
completely objective and accurate about your usual diet, food preferences, and meal pattern. The individualized diet plan that you formulate in Chapter 6 will only be as good as the information you provide.
For whatever reason, a number of research studies have shown that
overweight people are much more likely than lean people to underre-
port their actual food intake in surveys, diaries, and questionnaires. In
most cases I suspect this is unintentional, and may reflect a lack of
self-awareness of what and how much people are actually eating. To
minimize the possibility of underreporting, you should do two things
during your dietary assessment.

First, do not rely on recollections. You must write down everything
you eat as soon as possible after you consume it. Set aside a week in
which you know you will be following your usual eating patterns (not
during holidays or vacations, for example). Make your food record
from the day you start until the following week, not for the week just
ended.

Second, resist the tendency to restrain or "improve" your eating
during the period you will be recording your food intake. If, for instance, you sometimes grab lunch at the hotdog stand, it probably
won't hurt you to do that for another few days while you are recording your usual eating patterns. To get the best idea of your diet, you
should aim for recording a "bad" week rather than a "good" one.

One aside here, before continuing to a discussion of the behavioral
assessment, and that concerns the question of when you should consider seeking the help of a dietary professional. The answer is that a
professional is almost always going to be helpful, but it is not necessary for you to consult one unless you find that you are having difficulty tracking your food intake, or if your food intake records indicate that you should be losing weight, but you are not.

As noted earlier, there is a good deal of overlap and interaction between the different parts of a comprehensive assessment. This is especially so with the dietary assessment and the behavioral assessment. In fact, it is somewhat arbitrary to distinguish the two. For example, what we eat at a meal is a result not only of our specific food choices but also of our habits, environmental cues, and our emotional state at the moment. As you probably are aware, a "good" diet does not guarantee good weight control. It is possible to gain weight on a genuinely low-fat diet if portion size is not controlled appropriately. Thus, it is important to perform not only a dietary self-assessment but a behavioral self-assessment, too.

The Behavioral Assessment

All behavioral assessments at the Johns Hopkins Weight Management Center are performed by a psychologist with expertise in behavior change. If a psychologist or similarly trained professional is not available to you, or if you do not wish to consult one, you can use the questionnaires provided in Chapter 5, "Why Do You Eat?" to guide your behavioral self-assessment. In general, the aims of the behavioral assessment are as follows:

1. To assess your readiness for change.
2. To identify eating habits and eating cues that influence your eating behavior.
3. To assess your self-esteem, explanatory style, and coping mechanisms.
4. To identify eating disorders like binge eating, bulimia, or anorexia.
5. To identify and recommend treatment for depression, anxiety, or any other problems.
6. To integrate the behavioral assessment into your Personal Plan of Action.

The questionnaires in Chapter 5 are designed to identify your mood, your attitudes toward eating, your coping style, your eating habits (like binge eating), and other information that will enable you to select an appropriate treatment effort. In our weight loss center, this information is supplemented by an exploratory interview with the center's psychologist. This interview yields valuable information about the person's motivation for weight loss, past emotional traumas, the impact of the weight problem on his or her personal life, and current behaviors. I strongly urge you to consult a behavior change professional as you develop your Personal Plan. This specialist's insights and advice can be enormously helpful in developing a plan that is tailored to your specific needs.

The importance of this kind of assessment is clear in the case of Darla, a 41-year-old nurse's aide employed on an inpatient psychiatry ward who had been very obese since her early teens. She came to us because of a hip problem which would probably be improved with weight loss. She had never seriously tried to lose weight before. She related that her mother had been thin, and she had no recollection of her father, who was an alcoholic and left home when she was 2 years old. Her mother had remarried, and she had been raised by her mother and, from age 6, a stepfather whom she feared and disliked. At age 16, she left home and got a job. She later went back to school at night and became a nurse's aide. Although she had some friends, she had never been in an intimate relationship. She was in good health except for the recent hip problem. She had been prescribed Prozac once for depression but was no longer taking it because she felt she did not need it.

Darla's turned out to be a very complex case which is by no means typical of people trying to lose weight. Through the behavioral assessment it was clear that Darla had a number of problems that would interfere with her ability to lose weight. She was still clinically depressed, for one. In addition, she revealed that she had been sexually abused by her stepfather, apparently with her mother's knowledge. It seemed likely that she had gained weight at least in part to fend off her stepfather's unwanted advances, since he despised obese people. When she gained weight, the stepfather's sexual abuse stopped, but he became verbally and emotionally abusive toward her, causing her to leave home at a young age. Fortunately, the process of assessment helped Darla to deal with the aftermath of her troubled childhood. She lost only a modest amount of weight, but felt much better about herself.

While a good deal of information can be gleaned through a thoughtful process of self-assessment, there are a number of warning signs, discussed here and in Chapter 5, of problems that are best handled by a qualified professional, such as a clinical psychologist or a psychiatrist. If you have a past history or current symptoms of any of the following, I urge you to make an appointment with a psychiatrist or psychologist:

1. Symptoms of depression: chronic sleep disturbance; persistent feelings of hopelessness and helplessness; frequent crying; thoughts or plans of suicide.
2. Symptoms of eating disorders: frequent binge eating, with or without purging by vomiting, laxatives, or water pills (diuretics); wish to lose weight when already below normal weight; prolonged fasting; distorted body image.
3. Symptoms of thought disorders: recurring disturbing thoughts; hearing or seeing things that others do not; feeling that others are controlling you or plotting against you.
4. Symptoms of anxiety or panic disorders: intense chronic anxiety or fear; panic attacks.

If you have any of these symptoms, you will need additional help throughout your weight loss program, and you should seek it from a professional prior to beginning a diet. Getting help for any of these problems may have the additional benefit of making it easier to control your weight. Depression, for instance, will often sap a person's ability to sustain the kind of action required to design and carry out a good Personal Plan. Call your community hospital or a university center or your doctor or health insurance provider, if appropriate, and ask for the name of someone qualified to help you. To get the most appropriate reference, be sure to tell the person making the referral what you think your problem is—depression, eating disorder, thought disorder, or anxiety. Ask about the specialist's education (what degrees the person has, and where they were earned), and how long the person has been in practice. If you're not satisfied, ask for additional names—or you may be offered the names of several specialists to choose from, even without asking.

The Exercise Assessment

The term *exercise* has negative connotations for many people, but really what we are talking about is not just exercise but the full range of physical activity we engage in. It is rarely necessary to become an exercise "fanatic" in order to lose weight.

The aims of the exercise assessment are as follows:

1. To define your current and past levels of physical fitness and exercise tolerance.
2. To determine your usual patterns of physical activity and preferences for different kinds of exercise.

3. To measure your current resting energy expenditure via a test called "indirect calorimetry."
4. To develop an individualized plan for gradually increasing physical activity.
5. To set up physical activity monitoring for long-term maintenance.

Most of the details of the exercise self-assessment are provided in Chapter 7, "Exercise That Works for You." Some portions of the assessment, such as the indirect calorimetry test, you cannot do yourself. But you can do most of it. With the help of your honest answers to a series of questions, along with a willingness to try a variety of techniques to achieve your goals, you can make changes. Whether you are a "couch potato" or a "jock" or somewhere in between, finding enjoyable ways to increase your level of physical activity will make it considerably easier to achieve and maintain a lower weight.

When should you seek professional help to devise and carry out an exercise plan? First, when you have physical problems that make it difficult or unsafe for you to devise a traditional exercise plan. In that case, a consultation between your physician and an exercise physiologist, trainer, or physical therapist will make it possible for you to build an exercise component into your Personal Plan in a safe and effective way.

Second, if you experience difficulty in carrying out your exercise plan, an expert can guide you or even act as a personal trainer. This will help ensure that you follow through on a regular basis. Since such an approach is costly, I will describe a number of ways to improve your compliance with the exercise component of your Personal Plan—without having a personal trainer—in Chapter 7.

Finally, if you experience any chest pain, lightheadedness, severe shortness of breath, joint or muscle pain, or soreness as you carry out your exercise plan, you should stop doing your exercises and seek the advice of a physician and an exercise professional.

Comprehensive Assessment: The Synthesis

Once all the assessments have been completed, a staff member from our center meets with the client, in what we call a "synthesis meeting," to review the recommendations from each of the professionals who have performed the individual assessments. This is done after the professionals have met and agreed on an approach. Feedback from the client is important at this stage and may influence the plan that is ultimately adopted. The specifics of the weight loss plan are then discussed, and the plan begins.

In your case, the synthesis meeting will take place when you have completed the self-assessments and devised the individual ingredients of your Personal Plan. At this point you will step back to make certain that all the components (medical, dietary, behavioral, and exercise) are consistent with one another, and that you can carry out the plan that you've put together.

Here are some broad considerations to keep in mind for your own synthesis meeting. When you have finished developing your Personal Plan of Action and are ready to assess it, ask yourself the following questions:

1. *Is it comprehensive?* To be comprehensive, your Personal Plan must address *all* the major areas which can influence your success on the Plan, including readiness, physical activity, and maintenance.
2. *Is it realistic?* To be realistic, your Personal Plan must incorporate reasonable goals to be achieved through specific actions. You must be capable of fitting these specific actions into your schedule, and you must be likely to carry them out. If there's anything in your plan that you do not believe you can or will do, you should strike it from your plan and put a more realistic approach in its place.
3. *Is it permanent?* To be permanent, your plan must incorporate a maintenance plan, enough flexibility to respond to changes in your life down the road, and techniques of self-monitoring which will enable you to detect major deviations from your overall plan before they get out of hand.

Now that you have been introduced to the approach taken with patients at the Johns Hopkins Weight Management Center and have seen how you can adapt this approach to your own self-assessment, you are ready to continue. The next chapter describes the key ingredients of an effective Personal Plan, and guides you in developing your own Personal Plan of Action.

FOUR

Developing Your Personal Plan

So far in reading this book you have focused on understanding, and perhaps adjusting, your reasons for wanting to lose weight. By now you now have in mind several important reasons for wanting to lose weight. You have decided to do it for yourself and not for anybody else. And you appreciate the benefits of losing weight in a way that fits your lifestyle. You should also know that what you have set out to do is not easy, but this time you are going to do it right.

This chapter will help you assemble the tools you need for your Personal Plan of Action, tools to carry with you at all times. As you have seen, not everyone needs the same tools (which is why weight loss programs that try to serve the "average" dieter do not work in the long run). If your major problem is stress eating, you do not need to start calculating how much fiber to add to your diet. You need tools to help you deal with emotional cues and to put food in proper perspective. On the other hand, if you tend to eat only when you're hungry but then choose lots of fried, fatty, or sugary foods, psychological support may not be your most pressing need. Instead, you need tools to help you recognize what you're eating and to help you pick tasty alternatives.

Before you continue reading this chapter, make sure you have cleared away all distractions and have a pen and paper ready. Formulating a Personal Plan of Action is crucial to your success and requires your undivided attention.

Think of this chapter as a road map—a guide to the parts of the book that are most relevant to you and your situation. You can use this road map in two ways, depending on which of the following statements describes you:

1. "I haven't really figured out what my problems are or where to put my emphasis. Where do I start?"

   or

2. "I know what my problem areas are, and which ones cause me more trouble than others. But I'm having trouble doing anything effective about them."

If Statement 1 fits you, you are in good company—a lot of other people are in this situation, too. To identify your problem areas, begin your Personal Plan with a period of self-observation and reflection. Write down any associations you notice between what's going on in your life and what, when, and why you eat. You may want to go directly to Chapter 5 ("Why Do You Eat?") to get an idea of the habits to look for and the times when observing yourself would be helpful. During this observation period you should not watch your diet; instead, eat as you usually do. When you feel you have had enough time to step back and identify your problem areas, you can follow the steps described for Statement 2 with the additional advantage of having taken a fresh look at yourself first. You can only benefit from the insights you have gained.

If Statement 2 fits you, you're ready to read the next section, "Key Ingredients." This section will describe the strategies that all successful dieters build into their Personal Plans. If you omit any of these key ingredients from your plan, you'll make your job a lot harder. Include them, and you'll reap the benefits of others' success.

Key Ingredients

Build in maintenance from Day 1.

This key ingredient is philosophical in nature. Building in maintenance from Day 1 means that you understand, accept, and firmly believe that you are not going to reach your goals merely by going on a diet. You are going to build a Personal Plan of Action that will help you change your lifestyle and lead you with confidence into the next millennium.

What is the difference between a diet and a Personal Plan of Action? A diet is a series of short-term culinary sacrifices resulting in transient weight loss. It's an all-or-nothing exercise that many people have learned to do very well by practicing it frequently. It entails only two, mutually exclusive, forms of behavior: "diet mode" and "between-diet mode." In our society, people, especially women, but increasingly also men, learn this ineffective method of weight control as early as their teens or even childhood. They alternate constantly between the two modes because almost nothing is learned in the diet mode that can be carried over into the between-diet mode.

Your Personal Plan, in contrast, is really a blueprint for how you are going to live for the rest of your life. This does not mean you will be planning never to enjoy food again or to seek fulfillment primarily through running marathons. The idea is to make *gradual,* satisfying, and enjoyable changes in some of the ways you relate to food and physical activity—changes that you will choose and then want to make a part of your life for good. You will be justly proud of these changes and may even want to convert other people you care about to your new philosophy.

Set clear, reasonable goals.

We achieve our goals most easily when they are clearly defined and, more important, when they are attainable. Accepting a realistic goal is critical to long-term success—and to your self-esteem. All too often we see people who have so thoroughly bought into the false idea that thinness equals happiness that they set goals based on a weight they passed on their sixteenth birthday. This is a guaranteed way to feel like a failure. Don't fall into the trap of setting as your goal an "ideal" body weight. As we saw in Chapter 1, "ideal" weight is a misleading concept and should not be your target or your yardstick for measuring achievement or success.

At the Johns Hopkins Weight Management Center, we have adopted a different concept, one that has gained widespread acceptance among weight loss professionals—"reasonable goal weight." It is pretty obvious that if you have never been thin, you will be fighting a losing battle with nature if you make it your goal to be thin. You will do much better if you aim for the lowest healthy weight you have been able to maintain for one year or more *since* your early twenties.

Some of our patients, like many readers, may still yearn to weigh less than their reasonable weight. Clinging to this dream hinders rather than helps progress, however. To help our patients let go of this notion, we ask them to think about how much it would improve their lives just to get down to their reasonable goal weight, to remember the benefits of losing even more moderate amounts of weight (see Chapter 1), and to consider why so many people fail to achieve and maintain "ideal" weight. Extreme sacrifice can result in brief achievement of the elusive goal of thinness, but the cost is enormous and the achievement usually is only temporary. Some experts believe that un-reasonable goals can lead to lowered self-esteem and possibly more serious eating disorders such as binge eating and bulimia (see Chapter 5). Don't set yourself up to be disappointed. Instead, take pride in what you can achieve, and that includes more than just what registers on the scale. Your Personal Plan and a willingness to learn will put your reasonable goal well within your reach.

For those who still want to take off those last pounds, we suggest the following: use your Personal Plan to get to your reasonable goal weight and then let yourself experience life at this weight for six months or so. This will allow you to get comfortable with your abil-ity to maintain that weight. Then, if you wish, slowly reduce further. Under no circumstances do we recommend that people lose so much that they weigh less than their "ideal" body weight. We have had pa-tients at the Johns Hopkins Weight Management Center who say that they want to lose "just a few extra pounds" so when they "finish" di-eting they can eat "whatever they want" and still be below their ideal weight. As you can imagine, this is a formula guaranteed to cause rapid weight regain and yo-yo dieting.

Find a reliable support system.
A strong support network will help keep you on track for the long haul. Having someone diet with you is the ideal situation. The buddy system has been shown to improve the chances of successful weight loss. Probably the best buddy is a good friend or relative of the same sex who is enthusiastic, tenacious, and wishes to lose about the same amount of weight as you do. Your buddy need not fit this description to a tee, but you must be able to cooperate and support each other. Be careful if you choose a spouse or significant other as a buddy. In most cases this arrangement is loaded with potential pitfalls. Spouses and lovers may think they are being helpful, but they bring their own emotional baggage to the table, and it often gets in the way. Even though a sig-nificant other does not usually make a good buddy, he or she can be helpful by not making it harder for you (for example, by eating Häa-gen-Dazs while you are having a salad) and by being a nonjudgmen-tal, one-person cheering squad (for more on this, see Chapter 5).

What should you and your buddy do once you have found each other? The idea is not that you will do exactly the same thing at the same time. Your Personal Plans do not have to be at all alike. What is important is that you let each other know the details of each other's plans and understand what kind of support you need from each other.

One example of such support might be agreeing to talk with your buddy, by phone if necessary, any time you have the urge to do something outside of your plan.

Checking in on a twice-weekly (or, better yet, daily) basis with your buddy is also a good idea, for two reasons. First, it makes you accountable for your actions to someone you like and trust, someone who can both praise your accomplishments and encourage you after your setbacks. Second, it sets up a competitive challenge for each of you, since neither of you will want to report that you did not do as well as your buddy did.

Of course, competition can be a double-edged sword—it tends to make you lose weight faster, but it may also undercut the supportive aspect of the buddy system if it becomes too intense. To avoid this problem, try to focus any competition not on the number of pounds lost each week, but on the changes in behavior that are critical to long-term success, such as your new-found appreciation of healthier foods. Agree with your buddy at the outset that you will not discuss the specific number of pounds either of you has lost, and then stick to that agreement. That way, your buddy and you can both "win" in this competitive event.

Become invested in your goals.
A key ingredient in your Personal Plan of Action is the cheering squad. *You* are the cheering squad. We keep returning to the theme of knowing how to talk to yourself, how to cheer yourself on, for an excellent reason. No matter how good your plan is or how motivated you are initially, you will be unlikely to succeed in the long run unless you have faith in your ability to lose weight and you consciously remind yourself of the great reasons for doing so.

Though it might seem strange at first, we recommend that you actually say encouraging words out loud—things like "I really did a good job of avoiding the cake at that birthday party." How do you talk to yourself? Always be upbeat and positive, and speak with authority tempered by humor. Expect setbacks, but never let them get in your way. And never get down on yourself if you slip up. Remember, what you are doing is not easy, and you are still the same good person you were before that unfortunate encounter with the Boston cream pie. Be as patient with yourself as you would be with an infant who has to fall about 200 times before she gets the hang of walking. You are the infant this time around. Will talking to yourself really work? The short answer is—yes!

Most of us have had the experience of talking the wrong way to ourselves—and, lo and behold, the prophecies come true. If we were not incompetent, out of control, socially inept, fat, or whatever before we told ourselves we were, we became that way afterwards. Talking to yourself will have just this same kind of strong influence on you when you talk in a positive way. First believe, then you will become. We are not born with this high level of self-confidence. It is usually achieved through the effects of a stable and supportive upbringing and positive feedback in adulthood when we act in ways that show we believe in ourselves.

This attitude should not be construed as license to lose sight of reality and to unashamedly lie to yourself and the world. When you talk to yourself the right way, you can tell yourself the truth ("Yes, I slipped up pretty badly" as well as "I did a good job") and learn from your mistakes and your successes. Since you believe in yourself, there's no reason to hide the truth. When things go right, pat yourself on the back. When they don't, you will want quickly to correct whatever went wrong. To do that, you need to understand what happened and why. Then you will have the best chance of learning from experience.

To help you learn what to say to yourself in stressful food situations, read the following twenty positive self-statements.

1. Nothing tastes as good as having my weight under control feels.
2. I am in control of my eating; I can say No to any piece of cake.
3. Food cravings last only a few minutes. I can distract myself until the feeling passes.
4. Taking a walk is a good way to clear my mind, avoid eating, and relieve stress.
5. As a reward, I use praise, gifts, or quality time with friends instead of food.
6. I've been doing great on my Personal Plan, and I don't need to stray.
7. I have the strength to say No to poor habits and Yes to positive lifestyle changes.
8. I feel so much better when my clothes aren't tight.
9. I can get the tastes I enjoy in a fat-free substitute, and that's what I would rather choose.
10. To relieve stress, I deal with the things that are stressing me. I don't ignore the problem by eating.
11. I avoid situations that encourage overeating.

12. Social occasions are important to me because of the people who are there. The food is not the focus.
13. I eat to please myself, not someone else.
14. I eat in response to my body's needs, not my emotions.
15. I eat slowly and enjoy my food without distractions.
16. Fried, fatty foods are not as tasty as well-seasoned foods.
17. I eat only when I'm physically hungry, and I stop eating when I'm no longer hungry (rather than when I'm stuffed).
18. When I stray from my Personal Plan, I view the experience as a temporary lapse only. I get right back to my routine and try to learn something from the experience.
19. I eat at least three meals a day, including breakfast. This helps me control urges and eating in the evening.
20. I am nourishing my body and improving my health by choosing to eat at least five servings of fruits and vegetables each day.

You can memorize a few of these statements, or you may want to write some of them down to carry around with you; you can use them freely, whenever you want to. Add self-statements of your own that you find helpful. They can help strengthen your resolve. At the very least, they will entertain and distract you.

Make gradual changes.
One of the key ingredients in your Personal Plan is a technique you will see illustrated repeatedly throughout this book. It is based on principles of behavior modification, and it recognizes how difficult it can be for us to change habits all at once. Applying the technique of *gradual change* to your Personal Plan will make it more likely that you will permanently replace the old habits with the new.

For example, what do you do if you were brought up on whole milk, hate the taste of skim milk, but drink a lot of milk and wish to cut down on fat? Do you (*a*) hold your nose and swallow the skim milk, (*b*) limit your whole milk to one glass per week, (*c*) keep the whole milk and try to cut fat somewhere else, or (*d*) none of the above? The answer is *d*. None of the other solutions is very good. As we have seen, if you take solution *a*, it's likely that you'll either return to drinking whole milk or suffer with an unnecessary feeling of deprivation. Option *b* will also be seen as deprivation, and *c* constitutes a lost opportunity to cut down calories and fat in a relatively easy way.

Instead of choosing one of these unproductive ways of dealing with the situation, make the gradual change approach a part of your Personal Plan. Switch from whole milk to 2% fat milk. (By the way, this is a very misleading figure, since even whole milk is only 4% fat by volume, but fully *55 percent of the total calories* in whole milk are from fat. See page 146 for information on how to read food labels and not be misled.) While it may taste somewhat less creamy than whole milk, 2% should be close enough to keep you from feeling deprived. Use 2% fat milk for a month or so, then switch to 1%. (For an even more gradual change, you can mix equal amounts of 1% and 2% as an intermediate step.) You will notice something interesting at this stage. The whole milk that you used to prefer will now taste too oily. Taste preferences are complex, and they are changeable. Foods you liked to eat as a child you no longer eat; foods you wouldn't even taste as a child you now rank among your favorites. You can use the changeability of taste to your advantage in fine-tuning your dietary choices now.

Ironically, the fastest way to change is often the slowest, most gradual route. The same principles can be applied to other aspects of your Personal Plan, such as increasing physical activity and adding fiber to your diet. A side benefit of using the gradual change technique is that you can avoid the trap of endless sacrifice. Feeling that you are depriving yourself in order to lose weight sets you up for reverting to old habits, since no one wants to be deprived indefinitely. With gradual change there is little or no deprivation or suffering, only satisfaction, as the changes you've made become a part of the rest of your life.

Enjoy yourself.
You can enjoy designing and carrying out your plan. This will be obvious once you realize that you don't have to put things in your Personal Plan that you are going to hate. If, for example, you would rather listen to elevator music for half an hour three times a week than spend the same amount of time jogging, we will help you find some other way to increase your level of physical activity.

Not only will you hate it if you do something you don't enjoy, it will not work in the long run because it will never become part of your life. If you force yourself to do this unpleasant thing, you will resent having to do it, and you will drop the activity in short order.

Again, the concept of talking to yourself properly is important here. Ask yourself if there was ever a time in your life when you liked to do a particular physical activity—a team sport, for example. Then ask yourself what it was about that activity that you really enjoyed. Many people recall the camaraderie of being on a team as being a very important factor in their enjoyment of a particular sport. You may not be able to play a team sport regularly now, but you can recapture the joy of camaraderie by choosing an activity that fits your current lifestyle, such as exercising with a friend. Instead of telling yourself, "Exercise is boring," ask yourself, "What can I do to have fun?" It might be joking around with the neighbor while you play basketball, or seeing how many birds you can identify on a long walk (or interestingly attired teenagers, if your walk is at a shopping mall). It doesn't matter, as long as it is something you enjoy.

Don't underestimate the personal satisfaction of learning more about yourself and making positive changes in your life. Most people spend their adult lives locked into patterns they acquired in childhood, never to change. We all know the saying, "You can't teach an old dog new tricks," but there's another popular saying that is much more positive: "You're never too old to learn."

The personal growth you can achieve through developing and completing your Personal Plan is a wonderful reward. People often believe that if only they were thinner they would get the love and respect they deserve. The truth is, these things come with the self-confidence you achieve when you take control of your life.

If you think of yourself as someone who can't change, this is the time to practice talking to yourself the right way. For example, your Personal Plan may require that you change the kinds of foods that you eat. If you are trying to cut down on fats, you will have a hard time if you wrinkle your nose and say to yourself, "Foods don't taste as good if they're not cooked in butter," or, after trying a nonfat substitute for cream cheese, "It's pretty close, but there's nothing like the real thing." These statements are being made by the old dog in us, the part that doesn't want to succeed in making changes. Instead, try thinking, "You know, fried and fatty foods are not as tasty as well-seasoned foods, because all you taste is the grease, not the food under it," or, "This tastes like cream cheese, and I love the fact that I can eat it and not get all those fat calories." Try new foods, new forms of physical activity, new coping styles—they can all be enjoyable.

There are few greater sources of enjoyment and satisfaction than learning about and improving yourself. Remind yourself of this periodically, and take pride in your accomplishments. You will enjoy the process of change a lot more.

Be flexible.
The final ingredient in your Personal Plan of Action is flexibility. Your plan is not etched in stone. Though the plan is capable of carrying

you into the next millennium, it will only be useful as long as you build in flexibility, the capacity to change and adapt to new situations or changing needs. How do you build in flexibility? There are at least two ways. The first is to regularly reassess your needs and how your Personal Plan is addressing them. The second is building in back-up plans.

The plan that seemed perfectly adapted to your needs when you devised it may need adjusting as you carry it out. For instance, you get a new job with a new schedule and new stresses; you decide that you detest salads, which for a long time have been the major ingredient in your diet; or they close the local pool where you've been swimming for the season. If you have built enough flexibility into your original plan to absorb some changes, and if you are willing to adjust your plan, you'll be better able to deal with these kinds of situations.

How did some of our patients at the Johns Hopkins Weight Management Center deal with the need to change their plan? Bob changed jobs in the middle of implementing his Personal Plan, and in his new job he had to attend business lunches virtually every weekday to entertain sales clients. Instead of being able to bring his carefully planned low-fat lunches from home, he would be eating in restaurants. Since he had built flexibility into his plan, he was able to switch his lunch and dinner menus. He had his larger meal at lunch, allowing him to choose from a broader range of restaurant offerings (see pages 168–73), and he ate his low-fat "lunch" at dinnertime. As a bonus, he discovered that he felt less hungry when he got home after a filling lunch, and was less tempted to snack in the evening.

Sally put together the diet for her Personal Plan with a heavy emphasis on salads to provide fiber and bulk. About a month into her plan, however, she told us that if she saw one more piece of lettuce, she was going to start wiggling her nose like a rabbit. Because there is more than one way to cut down on calories and fat, she was able to substitute for the salads: now, instead of salads, she eats carrot sticks and broccoli florets dipped in nonfat dressing as well as some crunchy snacks like pretzels. This increased her satisfaction with only a slight hike in total calories. In the past, Sally might well have substituted potato chips or rich desserts.

Dawn loved to swim when she was a teenager and was excited about getting back into swimming as part of her Personal Plan. She joined her neighborhood outdoor pool and had a regular routine of lap swimming. She felt better and had more energy. Then the summer ended, and the pool was about to close for the season. What to do?

Join a more expensive and less convenient indoor pool? Stop swimming and lay down fat for the winter ahead? Dawn had built flexibility into her exercise plan by selecting back-up exercises. Expanding on the theme of enjoyable childhood activities, she switched from swimming to ice skating and rollerblading. Since she was not going to do these things as frequently as she had been swimming, Dawn also began taking a brisk walk around her office complex at the end of her lunch hour each day.

Even if nothing seems to have changed in your life, you should periodically reassess your needs to avoid burnout. You need to step back from your plan and see which components are working for you and which are not. This will give you an ongoing reminder of which areas you need to work harder on, as well as positive feedback for the areas you are handling successfully.

How frequently should you reassess, and how is it done? Ideally, reassessment is an ongoing process, but it helps to set specific time intervals for a formal reassessment, such as one, three, six, and twelve months after beginning.

What to Do Next

In this chapter you learned more about the key ingredients of a successful weight loss plan. Now you're ready to choose among the tools available in this book to develop a plan that's tailor-made for you, one that will help you lose weight safely and keep it off. To do this, first identify your problem areas in the list at the end of this chapter and check off the box next to each statement that applies to you. Next, on a separate piece of paper, write down the problems and the pages in the book that cover them. Now decide which problem plays the largest role in your weight gain and focus on that first, beginning by reading the pages of the book that cover your number-one problem area (many of them in Chapter 5 but also in Chapter 6 and Chapter 7). Remember, you do not need to fix every problem *completely* in order to succeed.

Take notes during your reading. Otherwise it's easy to forget what you have read. (We especially tend to forget the things we would rather not think about anyway.) These notes can also be used as a quick reference guide for you whenever you need a refresher course. When you have finished reading about the first problem, move on to reading about the next problem area, taking notes as you go.

After you have completed the checklist and have read and made notes on the appropriate sections in Chapter 5, turn to Chapter 6 to put together a low-fat, reduced-calorie diet that will be based on an assessment of your individual needs. Then go on to Chapter 7 to devise your personal exercise program.

Now you will put together your Personal Plan. It will be a plan with meaning for you, because it was designed by *you* to met *your* special needs. (To give you an idea of what to expect after the active weight loss phase, be sure to read Chapter 8, "Keeping It Off.")

Here is a sample plan, for Cynthia Fox, to give you an idea of how your Plan might be taking shape about now.

SAMPLE PERSONAL PLAN OF ACTION

For: Cynthia Fox   To begin: Today

Problem #1: "I eat when under stress."
Plan of Action

    A. I will identify stressful situations and keep a log of responses (ate/did not eat, distracted myself, substituted other responses).
    B. I will identify foods eaten most frequently when under stress (use log if not sure).
    C. I will problem solve:
        1. I will remove problem foods from easy access at work.
        2. I will bring nutritious, low-calorie snacks to work each day.
        3. I will make a list of what I need to do at work the next day to reduce stress.
        4. I will use the "watch trick" to remind myself to substitute other responses instead of eating when under stress (see Chapter 5).

Problem #2: "I eat too much fatty food."
Plan of Action

A. I will do a dietary assessment to identify specific problem foods.
B. I will try substitutes for the high-fat foods I am eating too much of.
C. I will monitor my fat intake for one week.
D. I will keep an eye out for new low-fat foods to add to my repertoire.
E. I will reassess my food intake at any time my weight increases by 5 pounds from my low weight.

Problem #3: "I don't have time to exercise."
Plan of Action

A. I will convince myself that exercise is crucial to my plan by reading chapters 2 and 7.
B. I will limit exercise to 20 minutes a day so it does not take up more time than I can comfortably spare on a permanent basis.
C. I will identify specific time slots that can be freed up for exercise.
D. I will schedule my exercise in an appointment book.
E. I will buy an exercise bike and place it in front of my television.
F. I will exercise at a fixed time every day so it becomes a habit.

A Few Final Thoughts

The "Personal Plan Ingredients Checklist" at the end of this chapter contains most of the areas you will include in your Personal Plan. The last four columns have spaces for checking off your regular reassessments. They are set up to occur at one, three, six, and twelve months, but you may reassess your plan on whatever schedule you wish. At the appointed follow-up time, ask yourself how you have done with that particular problem since the time you began your last reassessment.

Keeping a record or a journal can be very helpful in assessing your progress. For example, keeping an ongoing record of the date, circumstances, and outcome of each episode of emotional eating will enable you to see if the frequency of these events is decreasing, and whether you have been able to alter your response or at least change the kinds of food you eat when you are upset. Remember, for any given problem, you should not expect immediate or complete changes in longstanding habits. Use your skill of positive self-talk and the technique of gradual change to keep yourself motivated and moving in the right direction.

For many problem areas, extensive journal keeping is not necessary. Just do a quick mental check on whether you are making some progress in dealing with the problem. Either way, check off the box corresponding to the month and problem area after you have assessed your progress. Write yourself notes to document your successes, as well as the areas requiring more work or a shift in strategy.

PERSONAL PLAN INGREDIENTS CHECKLIST

Check			Book
Yes	No	Problem Behavior	Pages
——	——	I need help identifying problem behaviors	107–11
——	——	I eat on a rigid schedule	75–76
——	——	I eat emotionally—happy and sad	71–72, 76–79
——	——	I eat out of boredom	79–82
——	——	I eat when under stress	109–11
——	——	I use food as a reward	82–84
——	——	Food is my greatest pleasure	112–13
——	——	I pig out a lot	102–5
——	——	I'm physically hungry a lot	112–13
——	——	I binge-eat frequently	102–5
——	——	I eat many of my meals in restaurants	168–73
——	——	I eat too much in social situations	84–86
——	——	I eat too much in business situations	84–86
——	——	I eat when depressed	105–7
——	——	I eat while watching television	79–82
——	——	I eat while driving	76
——	——	I eat because it's there and so am I	97–100
——	——	I skip meals and restrain my eating	94–97
——	——	I snack a lot and don't watch what I eat	94–97
——	——	I need portion control tools	141–51, 163
——	——	I need junk food control tools	151–53
——	——	I need tools to control fat intake	125–29
——	——	I lack time to exercise	196–98
——	——	I hate exercise	190–92, 202–4
——	——	My metabolism is slow	175–77
——	——	Someone sabotages my dieting	86–92
——	——	I recently quit smoking	19–20, 92–93
——	——	Fat runs in my family	5, 44, 91–92
——	——	I don't believe I can lose weight for good	100–102

Directions: Answer Yes or No to each problem behavior by placing a check mark on the appropriate line. If you have answered yes about a particular behavior, place check marks in the last six columns at the appropriate time.

I Have Read	I Have Taken Notes	Follow-up (in months)			
		1	3	6	12
___	___	___	___	___	___
___	___	___	___	___	___
___	___	___	___	___	___
___	___	___	___	___	___
___	___	___	___	___	___
___	___	___	___	___	___
___	___	___	___	___	___
___	___	___	___	___	___
___	___	___	___	___	___
___	___	___	___	___	___
___	___	___	___	___	___
___	___	___	___	___	___
___	___	___	___	___	___
___	___	___	___	___	___
___	___	___	___	___	___
___	___	___	___	___	___
___	___	___	___	___	___
___	___	___	___	___	___
___	___	___	___	___	___
___	___	___	___	___	___
___	___	___	___	___	___
___	___	___	___	___	___
___	___	___	___	___	___
___	___	___	___	___	___
___	___	___	___	___	___

FIVE

Why Do You Eat?

Our approach to weight loss at the Johns Hopkins Weight Management Center draws on several fields of science and medicine, including behavioral science—the study of human habits, culture, and social interactions. Losing weight permanently, as we emphasize in this book, involves more than merely going on a diet. For most people with a weight problem, the "whys" of eating are more important than the "whats." In this chapter you will identify *your* "whys"—those behaviors that interfere with your body's natural ability to maintain a stable and reasonable weight. Through examples, you will learn to recognize inappropriate eating behaviors and to substitute effective ones. Sally is a case in point.

Sally is a 32-year-old single woman who works as a bank loan officer. She majored in home economics in college and is aware of the importance of good nutrition and healthful living. She can rattle off the caloric and fat content of many foods, and she almost always gets her "five-a-day" of fruit and vegetable servings (described in Chapter 6). Sally underwent a thorough assessment at the Weight Management Center, which turned up no medical problems, a normal metabolism, and an above-average amount of physical activity. Yet at 5'2" and 168 pounds, Sally was the only person in her immediate family who was overweight. Why?

Answering this question based on this limited amount of information about Sally would be difficult, not to say misleading. The reasons are many, and more complex than they appear. An important piece of information in Sally's case is that she had some habitual behaviors that contributed to her weight problem. One is that she frequently engaged in what we call "emotional eating." That is, she ate to excess as a response to both negative and positive emotions, under strain or when relaxed.

Food served the role of satisfying not only Sally's physical needs but her emotional needs as well. Perhaps related to this behavior was a pattern of eating large quantities of chocolate and other sweets during the week preceding her menstrual period. So, while it was true that Sally knew a lot about good nutrition, and generally ate a nutritious diet, her good nutritional habits were being undercut by her use of food to comfort or reward herself. Identifying the emotional triggers *in advance,* so she could substitute more productive coping skills, was a significant part of Sally's Personal Plan of Action.

At the Johns Hopkins Weight Management Center, we are surprised that more people don't develop a weight problem as a result of emotional triggers. Our culture encourages us to use food as a surrogate for other things. Few people overeat because they are physically hungry. When I ask a group of people who are overweight to tell me about the last time they were hungry and what it felt like physically, more often than not the response from the group is silence. Some people even eat when they are not hungry, out of fear of *becoming* hungry. The truth is, though, even for the poorest segments of our society, sustained physical hunger is not very common. There is malnutrition for specific nutrients, like calcium, iron, and certain vitamins, but caloric undernutrition is simply no longer a part of the typical American's experience.

We are bombarded with a staggering array of commercial messages advertising tasty (if undernutritious) food choices every day of our lives. These messages dovetail with an upbringing that, for many of us, included such rules as "Clean your plate, there are children starving in Africa," such comforts as "Here's a lollipop to make you feel better," and such rewards as "If you do your homework, you can have some brownies." Add your personal recollections to the list, and you can appreciate how many ways we have learned to misuse food and just how small a role hunger plays in when and why we eat. While thin people may also eat for reasons other than physical need, they presumably compensate for it later by undereating or through physical activity.

In addition to emotional comfort, food is often used in the following ways, usually inappropriately.

Food as habit:
> "It's noon—I guess I'll have lunch."
> "I should eat breakfast. I'll have a doughnut and coffee in the car on the way to work."

Food as comforter:
"A big meal at night gives me a pleasant, relaxed feeling."
"Food calms my nerves."
Food as pleasure or reward:
"After a hard day, I deserve a rich dessert."
"Food makes me happy."
Food as celebration:
"Let's go out to a restaurant to celebrate."
Food as boredom reliever:
"There's nothing to do. I think I'll see what's in the fridge."
Food as social facilitator:
"Come, visit, eat, talk, eat."
Food as entertainment:
"I love to cook, and I perform my own quality-control sampling."
Food as love:
"I made this just for you, because I care."
Food as art:
"It looked good."
Food as mountain:
"I ate it because it was there."

This is still an incomplete list, and you can probably add your own examples to it. The point is that in most of these examples, food is not really all that helpful. We are accustomed to using food in these ways, but not only is it inappropriate, it is often counterproductive. For example, using food to relieve stress may work temporarily, but let's look at it objectively. Let's say your boss puts pressure on you to do something unpleasant but necessary at work. It's upsetting, you don't want to do it, and you delay. You delay by taking a trip to the vending machines. You down a candy bar and diet cola, or even a relatively nutritious snack of yogurt and pretzels. You talk to whoever is near the machine. Soon the day is almost over, so you put off the unpleasant task until tomorrow. Perhaps you will fret about it at home tonight after dinner, and eat more. Needless to say, you are not hungry either time. Furthermore, the food has not helped you to deal with the stressful situation—in fact, it has distracted you from dealing appropriately with the problem. You may not even have enjoyed the extra food. You may not even remember eating it. And you still must do the task assigned by your boss. You have not solved the problem, only added another one—using food inappropriately, a sure-fire way to gain weight without really trying.

While changing your uses for food to a more natural, hunger-based system can be an important ingredient of your Personal Plan, we must be realistic about the feasibility of this approach, and its limitations. The patterns of food use described above are widespread. They are deeply ingrained in our culture, and in our habitual mode of behavior. They are indeed inappropriate, and contribute greatly to the problem of weight management, but they can be very difficult to change completely and to keep changed.

Also, recognize that correcting inappropriate eating cues is unlikely to result in immediate or substantial weight *loss*. This technique is most suitable for *maintaining a stable weight*, not for dramatic weight loss. That may be why few weight loss plans pay sufficient attention to it. Because regaining weight after weight loss is such a problem, however, we urge you to build behavior change techniques into your Personal Plan and to begin practicing them on Day 1 of your Action Stage. Then, after you have reached your goal weight, you'll already have countermeasures in place against inappropriate eating cues. Now, while you are still in the Preparation Stage and formulating your Personal Plan, you can use this time to observe yourself and learn more about your habitual ways of interacting with food.

Although behavior change without dieting is unlikely to result in significant weight loss, do not make the mistake of giving short shrift to the behavioral aspects of your plan. In many ways it is more difficult to examine your behaviors and change them than it is to complete even a very aggressive diet. The diet is wasted, I can promise you, if you do not address the behavior that caused you to gain weight in the first place (or to regain it if you have dieted before). *The opportunity to break this cycle of dieting and weight regain lies primarily in the effort you put into getting the most out of this chapter.*

Enough theory. If you have read this far, you probably are ready. If not, it may help to go back to Chapter 2, "Getting Ready," to convince yourself of your personal need to lose weight, and the need to change behaviors so you can succeed at managing your weight in the long run.

It's time to begin your self-assessment, using the tools developed by experts at the Johns Hopkins Weight Management Center. Begin this process with a positive attitude. There are few things more interesting to us than our own behaviors. Combine this natural curiosity about yourself and why you do what you do with the real opportunity to solve a problem that has been troubling you, perhaps for a very long time. You will see that it can be an educational exercise. An enlightening experience. A process you can even enjoy.

Behavioral Self-Assessment

The steps in this behavioral self-assessment should be taken slowly and carefully, with plenty of time to reflect on each phase. I recommend the following schedule:

Day 1. Read about people in situations leading to overeating. Complete the questionnaire, and reflect on the discussion.
Day 2. Read about people with various degrees of eating "restraint" and explanatory styles. Consider the questions and discussion.
Day 3. Read about a binge eater and people with other eating disorders. Again, consider the questions and discussion.
Day 4. "Visit" a depressed overeater (in this book) and people who also have mood and thought disorders. Complete the questionnaire and consider your score.
Days 5, 6, 7, 8, 9, and 10. Relax, step back, and observe yourself.

Day 1

Take a whirlwind tour of a variety of situations which contribute to inappropriate eating or to appropriate eating taken to excess. Your job is to picture yourself in each of the following situations and decide whether or not it is a problem area for you. There are only two rules: First, you must be completely honest with yourself. Second, if you are not sure whether the situation described is a problem area for you, assume that it is.

If you have absolutely no idea what your inappropriate eating cues are, or believe you don't have any, skip to Day 5 and begin a period of self-observation to identify a sample of your eating cues. Then come back to Day 1 and complete the questionnaire that follows.

Each question is followed by suggestions for how to deal with the problem. While it would be terrific if you could completely correct every problem area you identify, any steps in this direction will be helpful. Any positive behavior change will improve the likelihood that you will succeed in losing weight and in keeping it off permanently. Try to focus on the areas that are most relevant to your individual situation.

1.

Ivan eats "three squares" a day, without fail, like clockwork. He rarely snacks, but his meals tend to consist of large portions with second helpings. He may be hungry when he starts eating, but he will often continue eating past the point of fullness. "I guess it's just a habit," he volunteers.

Discussion: Ivan is engaging in ritual eating, that is, eating on a rigid schedule or in a stereotyped pattern. This is only a problem if it is combined with eating in excess of caloric needs. What should be done about a ritual eating pattern? If you believe you may be eating out of habit, when you are not physically hungry, you may want to try the following: For people who are on a normal daytime-awake, nighttime-sleep schedule, it is usually best to eat a nutritious breakfast such as those described in the next chapter. Do this even if you are not hungry. It has been shown in research studies that eating breakfast provides health advantages such as improved blood sugar control and better appetite control. It may also decrease the tendency to overeat later in the day.

For the specific habit of eating pastries, doughnuts, breakfast sandwiches, and other foods in your car while commuting to work, an effective tool is to plan ahead. Prepare fast, nutritious breakfasts the night before. Schedule this preparation time as a weekend errand. Buy fresh fruits, whole grain breads, jams or jellies, fat-free yogurt, and fat-free cheese and put breakfast-size portions in the refrigerator. Ideally you will get up 10 minutes earlier and eat these breakfasts at home. Or, you can continue to rush and grab a bag of nutritious car food on your way out the door. In either case, you will be less likely to eat the doughnuts, and may well find that your energy level is higher and lasts longer.

For meals after breakfast, do not eat automatically when the clock strikes 12 or 6 or whatever. Have a small snack of fruit, salad vegetables, or low-fat breads, crackers, or pretzels at the appointed eating time, and save the bigger lunch or dinner until you receive a physical signal from your body that you are hungry. You may be surprised at how much less food you will spontaneously eat if you are responding to your body's cues instead of clock cues. A caveat if you try this: Do not delay your eating times so much that you feel extremely hungry when you finally get around to eating. This can result in overeating, or even bingeing, later in the day.

2.

Maya is an emotional eater. Like Sally (described at the beginning of this chapter), she tends to eat in moderation most of the time but overeats in response to certain emotional cues. When she is feeling a bit "down" and alone, she consoles herself with foods that she usually would avoid. She may feel better while she's eating the "bad" foods (or eating "good" foods to excess), but she often feels guilty or more depressed later, which sometimes causes her to eat again. She is never physically hungry when she does this. Feeling down is not the only emotion which may lead Maya to eat inappropriately. She often responds to feeling anxious, stressed, or even happy by eating. She knows this is a self-defeating habit, but says, "The problem is, I don't even know I'm using food that way until I think about it later on, and by then it's too late."

Discussion: Many, many people have Maya's problem. Eating emotionally is one of the most commonly cited contributors to weight gain in our Center. For people with this mode of behavior, hunger is not part of the picture. Eating in response to emotions is a learned behavior; people are not genetically programmed to eat under these circumstances. In fact, most people who do not have a weight problem tend to eat less when they are under emotional stress. To see how strongly your eating is affected by your emotions, complete the following questionnaire on emotional eating.

Why does this inappropriate eating cue develop in some people, and what can they do about it? The antecedents of this behavior are not always clear. It is likely that you learned it from a parent or others close to you. This behavior is not directly taught, but is first observed many times in others, then tried, and then adopted as a habit. The reason it becomes a habit is because it is rewarding in some ways. If you are upset and you eat, you are distracted from whatever is upsetting by something that is genuinely physically and emotionally pleasant. Even for people without a weight problem, the process of selecting food, smelling it, chewing it, tasting it, and relieving hunger is certainly not unpleasant. And, as we've seen, food and eating are associated with caring and love in our society. The habit of eating in response to emotions is thus the equivalent for some of us to getting a hug or other form of reassurance.

Eating in response to emotional cues is okay except when it contributes to a weight problem. I call it "okay" instead of "fine" or "good" because, even if it does not contribute to a weight problem, there are usually better ways of dealing with an emotional issue than eating when you are not hungry. Recognizing that the eating response is not the ideal response is a prerequisite to kicking the habit.

What is the better response? Well, it depends on the circumstances,

EATING BEHAVIOR QUESTIONNAIRE: EMOTIONAL EATING SCALE

Do you have the desire to eat when . . .	Never	Seldom	Some-times	Often	Very Often
1. You're irritated?	1	2	3	4	5
2. You have nothing to do?	1	2	3	4	5
3. You're depressed or discouraged?	1	2	3	4	5
4. You're feeling lonely?	1	2	3	4	5
5. Someone lets you down?	1	2	3	4	5
6. You're angry?	1	2	3	4	5
7. You're about to experience something unpleasant?	1	2	3	4	5
8. You're anxious, worried, or tense?	1	2	3	4	5
9. Things are going against you or when things have gone wrong?	1	2	3	4	5
10. You're frightened?	1	2	3	4	5
11. You're disappointed?	1	2	3	4	5
12. You're emotionally upset?	1	2	3	4	5
13. You're bored or restless?	1	2	3	4	5

Directions: Circle the numbered answer that most closely matches your behavior. Add the total to get your score, and use the following information to interpret the meaning of your score.

Interpretation: For this scale, the average adult who is not overweight scores 17 (men) and 20 (women). Scores higher than 25 may mean that you have a higher tendency to eat in response to emotional cues than most people do.

Source: Adapted from T. Van Strien, J.E.R. Frijters, G.P.A. Bergers, and P. B. Defares, "The Dutch Eating Behavior Questionnaire (DEBQ) for Assessment of Restrained, Emotional, and External Eating Behavior," *International Journal of Eating Disorders* 5 (1986): 304. Nederlandse Vragenlijst voor Eetgedrag (NVE). Copyright 1986 by Swets and Zeitlinger, B.V., Lisse. Reprinted by permission of John Wiley & Sons, Inc.

and on your individual coping style. You are probably the most qualified to judge what to do instead of eating. Possibilities include talking to yourself, perhaps through a diary, about what is emotionally upsetting; talking to a friend or relative; or dealing directly with the source of the emotions, whether it be a person or a situation. For emotions or problems you are not ready or willing to deal with in the above ways, it is best to replace eating with another form of distraction, such as taking a walk, exercising, holding a pet, or even playing a video game. Just about anything will be preferable to eating inappropriately—try it next time and see. You may have to experiment a bit to find the best techniques for you. Having a flexible repertoire of alternatives to eating in response to emotions will serve you well in your Personal Plan for lasting weight management. If you are often sad, consider the possibility that you may suffer from chronic depression. You will learn the warning signs of depression on Day 4.

What about the problem Maya mentioned of not realizing that she is using food inappropriately until later on? This is a common problem. Even more common is not to realize that food is being used this way, even later on. There is a tool, called the "watch trick," which many people have found helpful in identifying and solving problems with eating cues. The watch trick is described on Day 5.

3.

Joe eats when there is nothing better to do. You might say he eats out of boredom. When he gets home from work, he settles in front of the TV and eats. If there's nothing on TV he wants to watch, he may find himself standing by the counter, eating a snack. He usually does this after dinner, but it also happens when he's home during the day. He says he eats because he's hungry, but upon further questioning he reveals that he does not experience physical hunger at all. He is eating because it is his habit to eat when alone.

Discussion: Eating when alone is a common pattern, and eating in front of the TV is a variation on this theme. With TV it is pretty clear why eating is a frequent accompaniment. A large proportion of the commercials are designed to put you in the mood for food. Unfortunately, your body may not need food when you are being urged to indulge. Also, commercials tend to hawk fat-laden convenience foods, perfect for eating on a whim when you are bored and not really hungry. This is particularly true in the evening when you may already have eaten a perfectly adequate dinner in front of the TV or elsewhere. When is the last time you saw fresh fruits, vegetables, or grains advertised on prime time? In truth, foods that should constitute the majority of our diet comprise a small fraction of the foods we are urged to consume through advertising. Why? Because staple foods tend to have lower profit margins than convenience foods and are usually generic—no one company stands to profit if we eat more of them.

I suggest you make a new rule in your home which says, "Eating permitted only in kitchen or dining room. No TV or reading material allowed." Make a sign featuring this rule and post it on the refrigerator and cupboard. (Note: diet drinks *are* allowed in front of the TV.) Other benefits of not eating in front of the TV: there's no mess, and you get to enjoy the taste of your food.

A word of caution: You have to be careful not to relieve boredom eating by substituting other food-related activities. Planning what to eat, preparing it, feeding yourself and others, making something new with any leftovers, then thinking about the next meal—all this can relieve boredom by taking up a good part of the day. We have learned to make all these activities enjoyable, rather than simply a necessary part of life. There is nothing inherently wrong with letting food become "something to do." It is only a problem when it leads to undesired weight gain or serves to reduce our motivation to find *other* satisfying, useful, or enjoyable things to do with our free time. It is also a problem if it leads to more eating or otherwise keeps you focused on food when you want to lose weight. This is the key to solving the eating out of boredom problem: *substitute something you find more satisfying, useful, or enjoyable for the food or food-related activities.*

The concept is to replace the easy, inappropriate response to boredom (eating) with an appropriate response. The specifics of the appropriate response depend on your individual needs and desires. They also depend on your willingness to try new things.

To generate a list of personally appropriate responses to boredom, take a blank piece of paper and make two columns, called "To-Do List—at Home" and "To-Do List—Outside." Make a list of the things you need to do (take out the garbage, return videotapes) as well as things you've always wanted to do (make a quilt, take karate lessons, volunteer at the hospital). Keep this list updated, crossing out things you have completed or lost interest in, and adding others as you think of them. Whenever you find yourself reaching for food when you are not physically hungry, look at your list and pick something else to do for awhile.

For those times when you are *extremely* tempted to eat inappropriately, it is probably best to pick something from your *outside* to-do list, because it will get you out of the house, far from temptation and boredom. Of course, you should avoid outside activities that are primarily food related, like going to the supermarket. Also avoid outside activities that include temptations to eat when you're not hungry—such as visiting your parents if they ply you with rich foods.

Usually, once you have gone and done your outside activity, the time for eating inappropriately will have safely passed. If you are again tempted when you return, it will probably now be an appropriate time for you to eat. You will have successfully converted an inappropriate eating episode into an appropriate one. Also, you will undoubtedly have spent your time more productively and/or enjoyably than if you had eaten out of boredom. Savor that accomplishment, and you will soon find it easier and easier to change your habit of eating inappropriately in this way.

When you are moderately tempted to eat inappropriately, when it seems like there is nothing more interesting to do, you should try something on your at-home to-do list. Here, you should also avoid picking food-related activities, such as straightening out the kitchen, and any other specific activities that often tempt you to eat, such as calling someone who upsets you. Food cravings usually don't last very long. Most people say 15 to 20 minutes is how long such urges last, so you don't need to complete a 1,000-piece jigsaw puzzle to get past the danger.

How about the specifics of your to-do list? If you are having trouble coming up with things, or even if you are overflowing with ideas, it can be helpful to subdivide the two columns into different categories of things to do.

Things that I enjoy:
    reading
    knitting
    walking
    games
    phone call to friend
    going to the mall
    going to the library
Things that are tasks but satisfying:
    straightening out sock drawer
    making a to-do list
    running an errand

Things that I have always wanted to do, or used to do:
take a class
swim
meet people
join a choir
volunteer at a school or hospital

Your list can be as broad as your imagination. Some of these activities can work really well to help you resist immediate temptations. The last category is not useful for immediate distraction but is critical in controlling the source of some of the problem, which is not being busy doing things you find enjoyable or worthwhile. You do not have to make every moment of your life interesting, but it can have a wonderful effect on your outlook as well as your eating behavior if you broaden your scope of activities, and keep your to-do list handy and fresh.

4.

Gayle believes she eats a fairly nutritious diet most of the time. At the end of a long day, though, she feels like she needs a little reward. In fact, sometimes it can become a bigger reward. She often looks forward to her food reward, thinking about it during idle moments and planning what it will be. Just the thought of it can cheer her up. "Food makes me happy. I really enjoy certain foods," she relates. Unfortunately, she sometimes gets a bit out of control with her food reward. These episodes do not qualify as binges (see later discussion), because she does not feel particularly guilty or try to hide her eating. Her eating-as-a-reward is not in response to hunger, though, and undoubtedly contributes to her weight problem.

Discussion: As with most of these eating patterns, using food as a reward, or food as happiness, is part of our culture, and thus can be difficult to undo. Perhaps it would be wiser to try and modify the response. That is, instead of rewarding or pleasing yourself with rich foods, are there other rewards that you can learn to enjoy as much? Alternatively, you could simply modify the ingredients and quantity of the food reward so as to reduce the impact on your calorie consumption.

First, though, it may be worthwhile for you to examine the whole concept of rewards. We use rewards almost instinctively as a way to induce ourselves or others to perform in desired ways. Rewards can be external (things like food, money, prestige) or internal (pride, satisfaction, a sense of safety or control). Generally, internal rewards are more effective long-term motivators. For example, a pay raise may keep you temporarily in a job you dislike, but you'd probably accept less pay and do a better job in a position where you were made to feel valued and respected.

The first question to ask yourself if you habitually use food as a reward is, "Reward for what?" If the answer is that you frequently suffer frustrating, unhappy days at work or at home, you may not need a food reward if you can make even a small, positive change in something that is making your life more difficult than it needs to be. It is impossible to guess your precise situation, but some general suggestions may be helpful. First, decide which things you can potentially change, and which things you are unable or unwilling to change. For those things you can change for the better, now is the time to plan it out, preferably in writing (for example, "I'll sign up for a computer course to see if I like that better than what I'm currently doing," or, "I will speak to my significant other about how much it would help if he or she did the vacuuming at home"). For those things you currently cannot or will not change, now is the time to accept them and plan more productive ways of dealing with less-than-ideal situations. (For example, "My boss's attitude is her problem. It's sad, in a way. Perhaps I should pity her instead of hate her.")

Identifying the sources of "hard days" and improving the situation can be a major undertaking, which may take some time to enact. Do not underestimate the benefit of even a small improvement in your hard day, though. Such an accomplishment is a powerful internal reward. It can prove to you that you can have a positive impact on your day, your eating habits, your food preferences, and just about anything else you set your mind to.

For dealing with food as a reward for good days (and as a reward for hard days you cannot or do not wish to change), modifying your response can be helpful. Make and keep a list of more suitable rewards. Use them instead of food. What constitutes a suitable reward is up to you. Some possibilities are a bubble bath, a small present (such as a magazine or a fuzzy pair of socks), a long distance phone call to a friend, a favorite TV show. The specific thing is not important and may be quite small. What's important is that you will enjoy it. The rewards you choose should not be used *instead* of eating anything. Instead, they are added to the reasonably portioned and nutritious meal you will eat when you are *physically* hungry. Although it may not strike you as much of a reward, a walk or other form of physical activity is in many ways an excellent "reward." This is because the emotional stresses of a hard day can be relieved very nicely by doing something purely physical. The advantage to this form of rewarding yourself is that it both relieves stress and increases fitness while helping you to lose weight. You can even get away with eating slightly more calories if you build extra calorie-burning into your day.

Finally, if all else fails and you occasionally continue to use food inappropriately as a reward, use the techniques of portion control and calorie and fat counting to minimize the impact of this habit and fit it into the fat and calorie budget of your Personal Plan. Instructions for devising this budget are given in detail in the next chapter.

5.

Carlo is a hard-driving, gregarious businessman who packs most of his extra weight around his middle. He never used to think about his diet at all, and never had to until the rude intrusion of a heart attack at age 51. He tends to eat a balanced, nutritious diet at home, thanks largely to his health-conscious spouse, but he has trouble controlling his diet in social situations, especially parties and business lunches. At parties, he can be found at the buffet table, inhaling huge quantities of rich appetizers. "I just like food," he states with assurance. As an afterthought, he adds, "And eating and drinking is part of my job. I have to keep my contacts happy."

Discussion: While Carlo's eating problems occur largely in business-related situations, many people report similar problems in purely social settings. It is known from experiments in which people's eating habits are observed that eating with others tends to increase the total amount of food consumed. This is called "social facilitation of eating" and applies equally to many animal species. It also applies to people who drink alcoholic beverages. The larger the number of people present, especially family or friends, the larger the meal consumed. On average, meals eaten with other people are 44 percent larger than meals eaten alone, even though the composition of the meal is about the same.

Social facilitation seems to occur in all types of eating situations—breakfast, lunch, dinner, and snacks; in restaurants and at home; on weekends and during the week. It might seem that a person who overeats socially could reduce the amount consumed by eating alone, but while avoiding social and business eating situations can be effective during the action phase of your Personal Plan, it is not a useful maintenance technique, since it would adversely affect the quality of your life. Also, as discussed in example 3, eating alone when bored may be a far greater problem.

There are alternatives: If you are hosting the event, you have a greater degree of control than if you are a guest. For instance, you may be able to have a very enjoyable party or productive business meeting that does not occur during a mealtime. Coffee and other beverages, preferably nonalcoholic, may be all that is needed. If the event does need to include a meal, because you control the menu, you can follow the low-fat and portion-control guidelines discussed in Chapter 6. As you will see, this does not mean that the food will be tasteless or boring.

If you are a guest, you still have a number of tools at your disposal which will help you to keep within the dietary guidelines of your Personal Plan. For instance, you can find out in advance what will be served. Even if you do not feel comfortable making special requests to fit your diet, you will at least know what to expect, and can plan accordingly.

If the food to be served is likely to take you off your diet plan, eat something substantial that is consistent with your plan just prior to leaving for the event. While having recently eaten is not a guarantee that you will not eat more, it will help you to maintain control. If you must travel a good distance to the event, plan ahead and bring food with you for the ride. If you are tempted during the event, go ahead and sample the foods you crave, so that you will not feel too deprived. Even the most fat-laden and calorie-laden foods can fit into your Personal Plan if you get the most out of a small portion by savoring it over a prolonged period of time. Choosing low-fat and low-calorie foods, however, will allow you to eat larger volumes and fill up earlier.

When your host or others urge you to consume more than you should, you may find it difficult to refuse. Depending on your personality, any of the following responses can be very effective:

Feigning shock:
"Are you trying to kill me? I know your delicious cooking. If I start I can't stop."
White lie:
"I already tasted it. It's wonderful."
Direct approach:
"I'm really trying hard to lose weight. I know you just want me to enjoy myself, but it's easier when I'm not tempted."

More humor:
> "If I eat another thing I will explode. It will not be a pretty sight."

Delay/distract your tormentor:
> "I'm just taking a break. I'll have some later"; or, "Where did you get this furniture? It's so comfortable."

Escape to the restroom:
> "Excuse me. I'll be back in a minute."

In business settings, sometimes the problem is how to refuse not food but alcoholic beverages. Try saying this next time: "I'd love to, but it puts me right to sleep lately"; or, "Thanks, but I'm going to save my calories for the entrée."

Perhaps the most useful way to learn how to deal with eating in social and business situations is to change your perception of the event. What is the primary reason for social or business meetings? Is the eating the important thing going on, or is it something else? Clearly the main reason for having a social gathering or business lunch is to meet with people you like, or at least wish to have like you. In other words, it is important that you recognize that such gatherings are primarily social or business events with food present, rather than eating events with people present. This may seem obvious, but our behavior often makes it seem like we are there primarily to eat. Instead, it is helpful to remind yourself right before entering the house or restaurant that you are here to catch up with the lives of your dear friends, or to make a good impression on a business associate, or whatever your reason is. Have a plan for the event, like: "I need to talk to Joe, Mary, and Bob especially." Focus on your party plan, and the food will remain secondary.

6.

Janet has had trouble keeping her weight at a reasonable level since she was a teenager. Many members of her family have weight problems. She was overweight when she married at age 21, but now, at age 32, she weighs 55 pounds more than she did then. She and her husband, Jim, have no children. Janet works in an office and Jim in a factory. She tries to watch her diet and recently considered buying a treadmill, but Jim objected to the cost, saying, "You're never going to use it, anyway. Just use willpower and stop eating so much." She is interested in lowering the amount of fat in her diet, but her husband insists on "meat and potatoes." He says he wants to help her lose weight, but he often brings home chocolate and candy bars. Chocolates are hard for Janet to resist, and she eats them when her husband is not around because she is embarrassed. Jim seems to be able to eat them every day as snacks and not gain an ounce. "I guess life's just not fair," she says, smiling weakly.

Discussion: There are as many variations on this theme as there are couples like Jim and Janet. The broad outline is similar—one partner has a weight problem and wants to do something about it; the other, who may or may not have a weight problem, is a saboteur. In my experience, the saboteur is often, though not always, the male; the "victim," female, unassertive and insecure. The saboteur may be genuinely concerned and willing to help, but he goes about it in a misguided way. Or he may *seem* to be concerned but actually enjoys his partner's struggle. Sometimes there is a bit of both going on.

Intentional and unintentional sabotage can be difficult to distinguish from each other. Bringing home rich desserts for a partner who has trouble resisting them, for example, can be a misguided expression of the "food is love" theme we've all learned, or a conscious or unconscious act of hostility. Other examples include:

Eating tempting foods in front of a dieting partner, relative, or friend.
Encouraging the dieter to "take a break" from the diet, or splurge.
Giving false sympathy:
"I don't know how you can eat that diet food, poor thing."
Giving negative messages about learning to manage one's weight:
"Aren't you hungry?" or, "Exercise is boring."
Giving negative messages about the dieter:
"You've tried this before; what makes you think this time will be any different?" or, "Why can't you just eat less?" and sometimes, "You're too thin" (assuming you are not) or, "I like you better heavier."

You need to learn how to recognize all these forms of sabotage, and how to deal with them effectively. To a certain extent, how you deal with sabotage will depend on the nature of the relationship and communication style you have with the saboteur.

First, how to recognize sabotage. You should observe, and record on a piece of paper, all episodes of dietary and behavioral deviation from your desired diet and behavior. Write down the date and time, the nature of the deviation, and what prompted you to eat. For example:

Date and Time	What I Ate	Why I Ate
5/6/96, 2:30 P.M.	Big piece of chocolate cake	Feeling upset with Mark; cake left over from Valentine's Day

This log will be useful not just for detecting sabotage, but also for detecting other conditions that derail your efforts during the action and maintenance stages of your Personal Plan.

Not all sabotage can be detected in this way. The subtle messages do not usually lead directly to deviations—rather, they undermine self-esteem and self-control. The verbal and body language can be detected by listening critically to your own feelings in reaction to these messages. Do you feel embarrassed by the other person's comments and want to hide your eating? Does something the other person says make you feel angry, or sad, or alone and misunderstood? Even if you do not respond negatively to these messages, you should be aware of their potential negative effect on your motivation for controlling your weight and adhering to your Personal Plan. You need to develop a way of dealing with sabotage appropriately, keeping in mind that the appropriate response varies from one person to another and one situation to another.

For people who are not important to you, you can simply recognize the hidden message behind such statements as "You're too thin," "Aren't you hungry?" and "I could never eat that way," and ignore the statements. You might even take some personal satisfaction in knowing that you are probably witnessing the saboteur's jealousy or insecurity about their own weight or eating habits. The statements are then unlikely to influence your behavior negatively, or distract you from the commitment you have made to your Personal Plan. If you are feeling insecure at the time you hear a sabotage line, the message can be more harmful, even if the person is relatively unimportant to you. For these occasions, it is particularly important for you to "consider the source." If it's your style to show no pain in public, you will want, again, to ignore the sabotage or just say "No" (that is, "I'm not hungry"). If you prefer the direct approach, you can say, with a smile, "Yes, I am hungry. Let's talk about something else."

For a person who is important to you, sabotage is usually better dealt with openly and completely. It is best to assume, at least initially, that the sabotaging words or deeds are unintentional. The saboteur may even be laboring under the mistaken belief that he or she is being helpful to you, that the statements or actions will motivate you in some way to stick to a diet. Thus, it may come as a surprise to the saboteur that you do not appreciate his or her "support."

Your primary aims must be to stop the sabotage and, if possible, to replace it with true support. Assume that your tormentor has good intentions and guide these good intentions into something useful to you. Start with a genuine statement of appreciation for the expression of caring and desire to help you in the difficult task of losing weight and changing lifelong habits. This is likely to be well received and may make the saboteur less defensive about your request for a different form of help. Even for the suspected intentional saboteur, this approach has much to recommend it. Only when the intentional saboteur does not respond to your reasonable requests and gracious assumptions of good intentions should you resort to other measures.

After starting with your statement of appreciation, what should you do next? This depends on the exact nature of the offense. An interaction might go something like this:

Janet: You know, Jim, I wanted to tell you that I appreciate how you want to help me to lose weight and keep it off.

Jim: Well, sure, I know how much it bothers you.

Janet: And you also don't get down on me when I gain weight.

Jim: Well, I know it's hard for you and it doesn't bother me.

Janet: Can I ask you to do something that would help me a lot?

Jim: Sure.

Janet: You know how I love chocolate and cookies and stuff; it's really hard for me to resist them, and they go straight into fat for me. You're so lucky about that.

Jim: Uh huh, but I just don't eat any more than I need; I just stop eating when I'm not hungry.

Janet: I guess I eat mostly when I'm *not* hungry, so it's hard to know when to stop. But what I wanted to tell you, since I know you want to help me any way you can, is that it would really help me if there wasn't anything around the house to tempt me for awhile. Will you take the cookies and stuff and maybe put them in your car, or bring them to work and only eat them at work or in the car? I know you like them, so this way you could have all you want without making it hard for me.

Jim: No sweets at all at home?

Janet: Well, I've got a deal for you. You know those sweet fruit fig bars that you sometimes eat?

Jim: Yes, but you hate them.

Janet: Exactly. Let's buy a lot of them. I really appreciate your help.

Jim: No problem. Hey, what's for dinner?

Janet: Well, while we're on the subject, let's talk about your meat and potatoes thing . . .

You get the best results when you know what you'd like the saboteur to do, and bring it up in a gentle but direct manner, preferably at a time separate from the incident rather than in the heat of the moment. This approach does not work in all cases, but it is worth a try. Notice how Janet defuses Jim's implied criticism ("I just stop eating when I'm not hungry"). Instead of rising to the bait, she concedes that she has a problem and goes right back to her plan of asking him to help her with it.

Sabotage does not generally end after a single such encounter, even when the encounter goes well. Because sabotage is usually habitual, good follow-up is essential. Just as you may struggle to change your own habits, the well-intentioned saboteur is also likely to slip back into his or her old habits. A gentle reminder, with humor if at all possible, can be effective. For example (wagging finger at errant spouse), "Are those my favorite cookies you snuck in the house? I may have to make you eat the whole box this instant, or else *I* will, and you'll have to feel guilty about it."

To avoid such potentially tense encounters, follow up your initial discussions with verbal reinforcement of your gratitude for the help you are receiving: "You've been really good about not bringing sweets home. I really appreciate it." Other possible reinforcers of your saboteur's good behavior include regularly sharing your success and delight with how your Personal Plan is going, praising the saboteur in front of family or friends, or giving him or her a hug, a small present, a note, or whatever seems appropriate to you. Don't hesitate to ask for help from your partner or others in your social network—only you know the best ways others can support your efforts to make lasting changes in your lifestyle.

For the intentional saboteur who is close to you, it may be reasonable to start with the approach outlined above. First, you may be mistaken about the saboteur's intentions. Second, even if you are correct, you may still succeed in changing his or her behavior, despite the initially poor intentions. You are basically providing the intentional saboteur with a face-saving way to change his or her behavior without blame.

If this approach does not succeed, and the sabotage continues, a more direct labeling of this behavior is needed. This doesn't have to be a hostile approach, but you must make it clear to your saboteur that you have pointed out the problem in the past, do not see a change, and find this puzzling and frustrating. Be prepared to hear some very negative things. When someone is accused of dishonorable behavior, he or she will often respond by attacking the accuser, rather than taking responsibility for his or her actions. You must not rise to this bait. Your requests are quite reasonable, and you must remain focused on them. The fact that your saboteur says he or she finds you weak-willed and contemptible is indeed an issue to be dealt with, but it is not your problem. He or she needs to come to terms with that kind of feeling, but it will more likely be resolved by supporting you than by sabotaging you. This is not an easy encounter, but it may need to happen for you to have a reasonable chance of carrying out your Personal Plan. If such encounters are frequent or unproductive, you may want to try couples counseling, which can do a lot to improve communication between partners.

You may choose to accept sabotage rather than deal with it directly. This is the only viable option in some relationships. In such cases, you must be prepared to enlist support from others—family, friends, colleagues—and to detach yourself from the nonsupportive person in your environment.

Finally, in dealing with the problem of intentional or unintentional sabotage, be aware of one very important aspect. The sabotage may relate to the underlying reasons for your desire to lose weight. It is common to want to lose weight because of a disapproving significant other. This is a negative, external influence, and not the best motivator in the long run. If this kind of influence forms an important part of your motivation, you must step back and rethink your Personal Plan a bit. Reread Chapter 2, and focus on internal motivators for better weight control.

One final note about families.

Your eating habits, as we have seen, tend to follow predictable patterns. They are embedded in other habits you may have, like watching television in the evening or buying a particular brand of bread. However, if you live with other people, your eating habits are probably not yours alone. Your habits are intertwined with those of your family members.

Families are about relationships, and psychologists define a close relationship as one in which important habits of the people involved are interlinked—the closer the relationship, the more habits people share. Say that your evening routine usually includes walking the dog, picking up the kids, and taking out the trash; think of the disruption that is caused when you go out of town for a week, just in the evenings alone. Now, imagine what will happen if you change your eating behavior *every single day, for the rest of your life.* You are likely to have a profound influence on the eating behaviors of the people close to you, and those people may react to the changes with anger and frustration.

We recommend getting the people you live with involved in your lifestyle changes. Without their help, change may be impossible. Studies of people with high blood pressure, for example, have shown that they are much more likely to take their medications when close family members are given information about hypertension and instructions about the patient's diet and medications. Your success at sticking to your Personal Plan depends on your ability to collaborate effectively with those around you. Getting your family involved in your plan may not be easy, but if all of you work together on this effort, you will make it a shared project and build a shared commitment to your weight loss. That doesn't mean that your family has to go on the diet with you or that they have to increase their physical activity. It just means that they should understand and agree to certain new behaviors like cooking without butter or excusing you from doing the dishes so you can exercise. In the end, the entire household will be rewarded with a trimmer, more vibrant you—one who will be around much longer.

7.

Ralph was always on the "husky" side, but he never really felt he had a weight problem until he quit smoking. In one year he gained more than 35 pounds. He is not sure why, since he doesn't really feel like he is any hungrier now than when he was a smoker. He has never been physically active and eats a moderately high-fat diet, but he has never been worried about his weight until this recent weight gain.

Discussion: For reasons that are not completely clear, most people gain some weight after they quit smoking. The average weight gain in the year after quitting is 6 pounds, but many people gain considerably more than that. The nicotine in cigarettes does increase metabolism, so there's a possibility that metabolism slows when smoking stops, but the effect is brief and is probably not the major factor in the weight gain, especially for those who gained more than the typical amount. An important and—fortunately—controllable factor is the tendency to use food as a substitute for cigarettes. Initially the mood-elevating effect of certain foods may help to soothe cigarette cravings in recent quitters. Later, eating may simply be a substitute behavior. Eating distracts the person and relieves stress the way cigarettes used to.

It can be difficult but it is not impossible to minimize the "bathroom scales" effect of stopping smoking. Here are some suggestions: First of all, change only one habit at a time. Do not try to lose weight and quit smoking simultaneously. For everyone but the morbidly obese, it is more important, from the perspective of risk to your health, to quit smoking than to lose weight. If you have quit smoking for more than six months, then it's okay to work on your weight problem.

Second, try to figure out whether you are, indeed, using food as a cigarette substitute; how and when you are most prone to do so; and what kinds of foods you are you most likely to employ. For example, for smokers, smoking after a meal is a common ritual. Now that you've quit smoking, do you substitute desserts or other snacks for your after-meal cigarette? Smoking cessation may depress mood, and some former smokers use sweets to elevate their mood or satisfy their cravings for cigarettes. Indeed, there is strong evidence that sweets do elevate mood, probably by affecting levels of a chemical neurotransmitter in our brains called serotonin. Eating small amounts of sugary foods such as hard candies or chewing gum can satisfy this desire for sweets without adding unwanted pounds. Try chewing gum after meals. While traditional sweets such as cookies, cake, and doughnuts are indeed sweet-tasting, they derive far too many calories from fat and are poor choices for a cigarette substitute. Better choices are sugar-free gum, crunchy vegetables, and diet drinks.

Third, to combat both the tendency to eat more and the mood-depressing effects of smoking cessation, try increasing the amount and level of your physical activity (see Chapter 7).

Day 2

Now that you are familiar with the common reasons for eating inappropriately, it is time to turn your attention to some basic behavioral concepts that may help you understand the ways people, including yourself, approach their eating. Here we will explore the concepts of restraint, self-efficacy, and explanatory style. As you did on Day 1, try to decide which concepts may be most important to you, and build the suggested actions into your Personal Plan whenever possible.

RESTRAINT

People's level of restraint in eating is graded on a continuum. It is not that you are either restrained or not restrained; instead, it's a question of how much and what consequence your level of restraint brings. We all have our own habitual levels of restraint which we must learn to deal with. Simply defined, restraint is the degree to which a person consciously controls his or her food intake. Luisa and Clara are sisters with different levels of restraint.

Both Luisa and Clara weigh about 180 pounds and are about 5'6" tall, but this is where the similarity ends. Luisa has been concerned about her weight since early adolescence, and has been on numerous diets. She has had some successes but inevitably regains the weight she loses within a year or two. She tries to be careful about what she eats, has learned a lot about good nutrition, and has adopted a low-fat, high-fiber diet—sometimes. She often skips breakfast and eats very little for lunch because she is trying to watch her weight. She reads food labels, and often refuses foods with a high fat content. Such vigilance drains her, however, and she has an unfortunate tendency to lose control of her eating in the evenings and on weekends. When this happens, she is often truly hungry because of the high degree of restraint she has exercised earlier in the day.

Clara does not understand how her sister can eat this way. Clara has never tried to control her urge to eat. It's not that she purposely eats to excess, but she always responds to her desire to eat. She has always eaten what she likes, when she likes, and in the quantity she desires, without giving much thought to the consequences—that is, until recently, when she developed some medical problems and was strongly advised to lose weight by her physician.

If you haven't guessed by now, Luisa exemplifies high-restraint eating, and Clara low-restraint. A fascinating experiment was done with high- and low-restraint eaters which illustrates the paradoxical consequence of high restraint. Subjects in a study were offered as much ice cream as they wanted under three separate conditions. First, they were told to eat all the ice cream they desired in one sitting. Second, the subjects were instructed to eat one scoop of ice cream (a "preload"), after which they were offered as much as they desired. Third, they were told to eat a preload of two scoops of ice cream, then offered as much additional ice cream as they desired.

The results? The low-restraint eaters, as expected, ate much more ice cream under the no-preload condition than the high-restraint eaters. After the one-scoop preload, however, the high-restraint eaters ate *more* ice cream than the low-restraint eaters, who felt more full after the preload ice cream and so ate less. After the double-scoop preload, the high restrainers ate slightly *more* than they had eaten after the single-scoop preload, and the low-restraint subjects ate even less.

How can we explain this?

The low-restraint eaters were responding appropriately to fullness cues, while the high-restraint eaters suppressed the urge to eat under the no-preload condition. But when required to eat a preload, the high-restraint eaters experienced "release of restraint" and ate more than the group that doesn't control their intake at all. This is the same phenomenon that many people experience when they stray from a restrictive diet. Once they stray, they figure, "Well, I blew it, so I might as well eat the rest of this cheesecake." Clearly, this response is inappropriate. The lesson here is that when it comes to restraint, *moderation is the key.*

How can this understanding of restraint help you achieve a good balance? First, look at the pattern of your own eating. Is it closer to Luisa's or to Clara's? The Restraint Scale (below) can help you answer this question. If you are a restrained eater like Luisa, you may need to loosen your restraint a bit (we will discuss how below). If you are an unrestrained eater like Clara, you may want to impose some restraints on the situations or habits that have contributed to weight gain. Recognize also that few people are pure Luisa or pure Clara. There may be times when you are highly restrained and other times when you exercise no restraint. Probably the most useful way to use your understanding of restraint is to analyze each situation that comes up with restraint in mind. Then consciously decide how much restraint is appropriate.

As with most behaviors, though, our restraint (or lack of it) is recognized most readily in retrospect. What was your immediate response to the question of whether your eating patterns are most like Luisa's (restrained) or like Clara's (unrestrained)? If you feel that you are overly restrained, it is time to look at the pattern of your daily food intake. Do you eat mostly in the evening, or do you spread your meals evenly? If you tend to consume most of your calories later in the day, eating a bigger breakfast or lunch or enjoying a midmorning

EATING BEHAVIOR QUESTIONNAIRE: RESTRAINT SCALE

	Never	Seldom	Some- times	Often	Very Often
1. When you have put on weight, do you eat less than you usually do?	1	2	3	4	5
2. Do you try to eat less at meal- times than you would like to eat?	1	2	3	4	5
3. How often do you refuse food or drink offered you because you are concerned about your weight?	1	2	3	4	5
4. Do you watch exactly what you eat?	1	2	3	4	5
5. Do you deliberately eat foods that are not fattening?	1	2	3	4	5
6. When you have eaten too much, do you subsequently eat less to avoid becoming heavier?	1	2	3	4	5
7. Do you deliberately eat less to avoid becoming heavier?	1	2	3	4	5
8. How often do you try not to eat between meals because you are watching your weight?	1	2	3	4	5
9. How often in the evenings do you try not to eat because you are watching your weight?	1	2	3	4	5
10. Do you take your weight into account in deciding what to eat?	1	2	3	4	5

Directions: Circle the numbered answer that most closely matches your behavior. Add the total to get your score, and use the following information to interpret the meaning of your score.

Interpretation: For this scale, the average adult who is not overweight scores 18 (men) and 24 (women). A score of 30 is usual for overweight women. If you scored higher than 35, this suggests that you exercise a high degree of restraint over your eating.

Source: Adapted from T. Van Strien, J.E.R. Frijters, G.P.A. Bergers, and P. B. Defares, "The Dutch Eating Behavior Questionnaire (DEBQ) for Assessment of Restrained, Emotional, and External Eating Behavior," *International Journal of Eating Disorders* 5 (1986): 304. Nederlandse Vragenlijst voor Eetgedrag (NVE). Copyright 1986 by Swets and Zeitlinger, B.V., Lisse. Reprinted by permission of John Wiley & Sons, Inc.

or midafternoon snack may be useful. Most people's energy needs are highest during the early and middle portions of the day anyway, so that's when your body can make best use of the energy produced by food. If you make this switch to less restraint earlier in the day, you will be less likely to overeat late in the day or evening.

The highly restrained eater is also likely to pass up favorite foods entirely, leading to feelings of deprivation later and loss of control. Try using tasty substitutes for favorite foods (for example, substitute a moderate-sized portion of fat-free and sugar-free frozen yogurt for premium chocolate ice cream), or use small portions of favorite foods. This can help prevent problems late in the day.

The unrestrained eater, on the other hand, may benefit from a period of self-monitoring, or keeping a food diary (see Chapter 6 for information about this tool). Learning about portion sizes and how to control portions (also in Chapter 6) is also useful for this person. The idea is to achieve a moderate level of restraint for both the unrestrained and the highly restrained eater. This means exercising restraint every time you eat, but being aware of your physical and emotional needs.

EXPLANATORY STYLE AND SELF-ESTEEM

Another important influence on your eating behaviors is your explanatory style. Recognizing that few people are all one way or all the other way, we can still find it useful for our discussion to divide people into two general categories of explanatory style.

The first type of person tends to explain life in terms of external, hard-to-influence forces. They answer the question, "Why haven't I been able to lose weight?" with reasons like "Because the world conspires against me—the stresses of my life, my unsupportive family, my job and the long hours"; or, "My metabolism must be off, because I can just smell a piece of cake and gain weight"; or, "I just can't exercise because I don't have the time, and besides, no one has explained to me what kind of exercise to do"; or, "I just can't resist things that taste good, even if I'm not hungry." Psychologists call this explanatory style "external locus of control" or "external" for short. It means the tendency to explain problems in terms of forces, places, or people which are largely outside your personal control.

The second style, as you may have guessed, explains life in terms of internal, controllable forces. For such individuals, the same question, "Why haven't I been able to lose weight?" produces this kind of answer: "Because I have not stuck with what I intended to do. The stresses of my life do not make it any easier, but I need to see if I can reduce them, or work around them. If my metabolism is slow, I should find out whether this can be offset by eating differently or exercising more."

While few people exclusively use one or the other explanatory style, you probably have a sense of how you usually respond to problems. To see how you rate when it comes to responding to external eating cues, complete the External Eating Questionnaire (below). There are pros and cons to each kind of response. Certainly, if there is a problem you truly can do nothing about, it is not helpful to approach it as something you believe you should be able to fix. An example of this might be a co-worker who dislikes you because of your religion or your race. While you may need to co-exist with this person, believing that you can change your co-worker's opinion by behaving a certain way, or that you are somehow responsible for their opinion, is probably less desirable than simply saying, "It's not my fault, he's just prejudiced and insecure."

On the other hand, if the problem is that you haven't been able to lose weight, the external style is probably not going to result in long-term behavior change. The external explanatory style allows you to make excuses for your current situation, and for not trying to change. The internal explanatory style is best for successful weight loss, because it puts the responsibility squarely within you—you are the person who can make this work.

The only potential drawback to an internal explanatory style in weight management is the tendency to be too hard on yourself when things do not go perfectly. Those who employ the internal explanatory style may blame themselves for everything and view anything less than unqualified success as a kind of failure. This belief is all the more damaging because of the notion that it is due to a personal failing—a lack of strength, perhaps. While it is probably best not to blame the outside world when weight loss doesn't proceed according to your Personal Plan, it is also best to keep the problem in perspective and not blame yourself entirely. That is, accept responsibility for small and large deviations from your plan, but don't dwell on them or attribute them to giant failings in your character. For example, it is useful to accept that your actions at the party resulted in an estimated 1,000-calorie deviation from your plan and erased three days of stellar adherence; it is not useful to conclude that you are a bad person who is not capable of change.

EATING BEHAVIOR QUESTIONNAIRE: EXTERNAL SCALE

	Never	Seldom	Some-times	Often	Very Often
1. If food tastes good to you, do you eat more than usual?	1	2	3	4	5
2. If food smells and looks good, do you eat more than usual?	1	2	3	4	5
3. If you see or smell something delicious, do you have a desire to eat it?	1	2	3	4	5
4. If you have something delicious to eat, do you eat it right away?	1	2	3	4	5
5. If you walk past the bakery, do you have the desire to buy something delicious?	1	2	3	4	5
6. If you walk past a snack bar or a cafe, do you have the desire to buy something delicious?	1	2	3	4	5
7. If you see others eating, do you have the desire to eat?	1	2	3	4	5
8. Can you resist eating delicious foods?	5	4	3	2	1
9. Do you eat more than usual when you see others eating?	1	2	3	4	5
10. When preparing a meal, are you inclined to eat something?	1	2	3	4	5

Directions: Circle the numbered answer that most closely matches your behavior. Add the total to get your score, and use the following information to interpret the meaning of your score.

Interpretation: For this scale, the average adult who is not overweight scores 26 (men) and 27 (women). If you scored higher than 35, this suggests that you respond more than most people to external eating cues.

Source: Adapted from T. Van Strien, J.E.R. Frijters, G.P.A. Bergers, and P. B. Defares, "The Dutch Eating Behavior Questionnaire (DEBQ) for Assessment of Restrained, Emotional, and External Eating Behavior," *International Journal of Eating Disorders* 5 (1986): 304. Nederlandse Vragenlijst voor Eetgedrag (NVE). Copyright 1986 by Swets and Zeitlinger, B.V., Lisse. Reprinted by permission of John Wiley & Sons, Inc.

If you tend toward the external explanatory style, it can be helpful to start examining your thinking and see whether you can reframe your approach a bit, at least as it applies to weight loss. For example, if you find yourself thinking that a food problem is outside your control, or that you cannot change a particular eating behavior, ask yourself whether this really is so. Perhaps you just need to develop a new strategy for dealing with it. This book is full of strategies and tools that address specific problem areas. If you pick and choose the most relevant ones for your situation, your Personal Plan of Action will help you prove to yourself that you are in control, and that it is usually not necessary to blame others.

SELF-EFFICACY AND SELF-ESTEEM

Self-efficacy is the belief that you can make specific changes in your life. Weight management self-efficacy, then, is the belief that you can manage your weight effectively. Self-esteem is a broader, less well-defined concept concerning your estimation of your own worth as a person. Many people confuse these concepts, but it's very useful to maintain the distinction between them. While the level of self-efficacy is usually similar to the level of self-esteem, this is not always the case. A person can have low self-efficacy and high self-esteem, or vice versa, and any gradation in between. This means that even a person who has high self-esteem may believe that losing weight is beyond his or her control. Or, a person can have generally low self-esteem but still believe that controlling weight is within his or her power.

We find that many people with weight problems suffer from low self-esteem and low self-efficacy, but we are not sure why this is so. It is clear that society's prejudices contribute to the low self-esteem of many obese persons. But it is probably not true that low self-esteem *causes* weight problems. Low weight management self-efficacy, on the other hand, in an individual who is genetically or environmentally susceptible to excessive weight gain, will make it far more difficult for that person to control his or her weight. Even if your self-esteem is high, you may have learned through experience that you are generally unsuccessful at maintaining a stable, healthy weight. This contributes to even lower self-efficacy in a continuous downward spiral.

While the evidence is scant, it also makes sense that continued lack of success in weight control may adversely affect your general level of self-esteem. Obviously, both of these consequences are undesirable. Lack of weight management self-efficacy and low self-esteem jeopardize the outcome of a weight control plan in a phenomenon called a "self-fulfilling prophecy." In other words, if you don't believe that you can be successful, you won't be. And, if you are initially successful despite a lack of belief in your own abilities, the success may be jeopardized by negative thinking such as: "It can't be true. I'm going to mess it up somehow." When the first signs of relapse occur, they may be greeted almost with relief, because relapse is the expected outcome for the person burdened with low self-efficacy or low self-esteem.

If your self-efficacy with regard to weight control is low, is there anything you can do to improve it? Yes. You can change your mind-set. If you develop a belief in your ability to achieve and maintain a healthy weight, and combine that belief with the proper tools, your chances of success will be vastly improved.

How can you adopt a more positive mind-set? First, do things that require no change in mind-set but will establish the conditions for success. These include recognizing appropriate motivators and having a coherent plan. Thus, the first step in improving your level of self-efficacy with regard to successful weight management is to finish reading this book and, in the process, develop your Personal Plan of Action.

Next, you must begin to pay attention to your successes, no matter how small. Let's assume for the moment that your weight management self-efficacy is about as low as it can be. Even at this minimal level of confidence, there is always some positive experience to build on in the path to successful weight management. Think back over the past decade or two: Was there any time when you achieved a modicum of success at maintaining a stable, healthy weight, even if it was very brief? If so, you have proved that you *can* do it.

What were you doing correctly at that time? How is it that you were able to do it then? Can you reinstitute at least one of the conditions that enabled you to be successful in the past? Perhaps you were more physically active, or your stress was under better control, or you believed in your ability more at that time. A change of mind-set can often be achieved by recalling past successes and applying some of the same attitudes to the present.

Even when there is no past success to build on, there are examples of desirable behaviors that serve the same purpose. For example, if you have a craving for a specific food (chocolate cake), or have a tendency to eat to excess under a specific condition (for example, your mother's telephone calls upset you), can you think of the last time you did *not* eat the entire chocolate cake, or did not eat but instead got out of the house to clear your mind? You almost certainly can think of such an occasion.

Write down the specifics of the occasion below:

_____

_____

_____

What you'll find is that there are times when you *are* able to stop eating chocolate cake before you are stuffed, or do something other than eat in response to emotional stress. Your job now is to recognize and accept this ability, to analyze what you did *right* and build on it.

Over the next ten times the temptation or stress occurs, perhaps you can aim for the modest goal of behaving in a successful way one time out of ten. As you know, if you can do it one of the ten times, you can surely do it two out of ten times. Pay attention to what you do right, mimic it, and improve on it. Pretty soon you will have yourself believing that you can do it right three or four or even nine out of ten times. Even if you do only slightly better than you used to, this is important—you must recognize that it is important and give yourself credit. Your weight may not change significantly from small changes in mind-set, but building on effective, successful behaviors is in fact very important for maintaining a new, lower weight.

The third phase in improving your mind-set about weight management is to learn how to talk to yourself. As discussed in Chapter 4, a key ingredient for success is learning to be your own best booster. Some people are already good at this, but many people, unfortunately, have learned instead to be their own harshest critic. The causes of this maladaptive attitude are various. They include excessively high personal expectations, negative childhood experiences, and self-protection. The causes really don't matter as much as the fact that such an attitude doesn't get people very far toward their goals in life. The old concept of a self-fulfilling prophecy comes into play when we are overly self-critical and predict our own failure.

The best way to change how you talk to yourself is to just do it. Remarkable as it may seem, just saying positive things to yourself will ultimately silence the critical voice within. Learn to give yourself a break, and you will lift a great burden from your shoulders. You may even improve your self-efficacy, self-esteem, and weight control.

Day 3

Today we will visit with Alice-Ann. Alice-Ann is very conscious of her weight. She was never very overweight, but she comes from a family where being thin was important. She gained weight after her daughter was born and she quit her job as an office clerk. She is a very restrained eater, and rarely eats much around other people. Several times a week, however, she binges. These binges are not the same as what we have previously described as simple overeating. What Alice-Ann does is eat, in a couple of hours, much more food than normal, while alone at home. She feels as if she cannot stop eating, and then feels guilty or sad afterwards. She is very afraid, both of the binges and of gaining more weight. She is currently 190 pounds and stands 5'5" tall. Alice-Ann came to the Johns Hopkins Weight Management Center for help in losing weight. As part of her assessment, she was given the following questionnaire. If you see some aspects of yourself in Alice-Ann, complete the questionnaire below.

BINGE SCALE QUESTIONNAIRE

Binge eating is defined as the rapid consumption of a large quantity of food, usually within less than two hours. Often a person who binges feels out of control, fearing that he or she will not be able to stop eating. Once the binge ends, that person often feels guilty and depressed.

1. How often do you binge eat?
   A. Seldom
   B. Once or twice a month
   C. Once a week
   D. Almost every day
2. What is the average length of an eating episode?
   A. Less than 15 minutes
   B. 15 minutes to an hour
   C. 1 to 4 hours
   D. More than 4 hours
3. Which of the following statements best applies to your binge eating?
   A. I eat until I have had enough to satisfy me.
   B. I eat until my stomach feels full.
   C. I eat until my stomach is painfully full.
   D. I eat until I can't eat anymore.
4. Do you ever vomit after a binge?
   A. Never
   B. Sometimes
   C. Usually
   D. Always

BINGE SCALE QUESTIONNAIRE (Cont.)

5. Which of the following statements best applies to your eating
   behavior when binge eating?
   A. I eat more slowly than usual.
   B. I eat about the same way as I usually do.
   C. I eat very rapidly.
6. How much are you concerned about your binge eating?
   A. Not bothered at all
   B. Bothers me a little
   C. Moderately concerned
   D. A major concern
7. Which of the following statements best describes your feelings
   during a binge?
   A. I feel that I could control the eating if I chose.
   B. I feel that I have at least some control.
   C. I feel completely out of control.
8. Which of the following statements describes your feelings after
   a binge?
   A. I feel fairly neutral, not too concerned.
   B. I am moderately upset.
   C. I hate myself.
9. Which of the following phrases most accurately describes your
   feelings after a binge?
   A. Not depressed at all
   B. Mildly depressed
   C. Moderately depressed
   D. Very depressed

Scoring: The questionnaire helps distinguish people who meet criteria for
binge eating from people who do not, even if they occasionally binge eat.
While an expert is required to make a diagnosis, you should be aware that
you may have an eating disorder if you answered the above questions in
the following manner:

1. c or d
2. b, c, or d
3. c or d
4. b, c, or d may indicate bulimia nervosa (see below)
5. usually c
6. c or d
7. b or c
8. b or c
9. b, c, or d

Source: R. C. Hawkins and P. Clement, "Development and Construct Validation of a Self-report
Measure of Binge Eating Tendencies," *Addictive Behaviors* 5 (1980): 219–26. Reprinted by permission of Elsevier Science Ltd., Oxford, England.

In brief, binge-eating disorder is defined by having two or more episodes per week of binge eating: a distinct episode of excessive, rapid food consumption, in private, which you are unable to stop, accompanied or followed by a negative emotional state like sadness, anger, or guilt. If you feel you may meet these criteria for binge-eating disorder, you are not alone. Studies of overweight women who see a doctor for treatment, for example, suggest that up to 30 percent meet the criteria for a diagnosis of this eating disorder.

If you have binge-eating disorder, you need to seek professional help from a psychologist or psychiatrist skilled in the treatment of eating disorders. While it is beyond the scope of this book to detail the techniques used in treatment, successful treatment does exist. Some of the techniques used by experts include stimulus control, cognitive and interpersonal therapy, and sometimes medications. While the Personal Plan you are building will be helpful to you, you will only succeed if you also seek the in-person opinion of an expert about this particular problem.

If binge-eating disorder is accompanied by attempts to rid the body of the excessive food, it is called bulimia nervosa. People with bulimia nervosa may use laxatives, diuretics, or vomiting to purge (Question 4), as well as fasting or excessive exercise. Binge eating, with or without bulimia nervosa, can seriously affect your health. You need to seek help, and I urge you to do so.

Day 4

Today you will assess yourself for a condition that can affect your perception of the world and your life, as well as your ability to develop and adhere to a Personal Plan: depression. As mentioned earlier in the chapter, depression is common among people with weight problems or eating disorders, regardless of whether it predates or follows weight gain. The symptoms and signs of depression include some things you might expect (such as crying spontaneously) along with others that you might not, such as change in appetite and waking up early in the morning.

The Depression Questionnaire (below) is often used as part of an evaluation to determine whether someone is suffering from this condition. It was developed in 1975 by the Center for Epidemiologic Studies at the National Institutes of Health. Circle your honest response to each of the following questions, even if you do not think you are depressed. Depression is almost always treatable, and it is a

DEPRESSION QUESTIONNAIRE

During the past week:	Rarely or None of the Time (Less Than 1 Day)	Some or Little of the Time (1–2 Days)	Occasionally or a Moderate Amount of Time (3–4 Days)	Most or All of the Time (5–7 Days)
1. I was bothered by things that usually don't bother me	0	1	2	3
2. I did not feel like eating; my appetite was poor	0	1	2	3
3. I felt that I could not shake off the blues, even with help from my family or friends	0	1	2	3
4. I felt that I was just as good as other people	3	2	1	0
5. I had trouble keeping my mind on what I was doing	0	1	2	3
6. I felt depressed	0	1	2	3
7. I felt that everything I did was an effort	0	1	2	3
8. I felt hopeful about the future	3	2	1	0
9. I thought my life had been a failure	0	1	2	3
10. I felt fearful	0	1	2	3
11. My sleep was restless	0	1	2	3
12. I was happy	3	2	1	0
13. I talked less than usual	0	1	2	3
14. I felt lonely	0	1	2	3
15. People were unfriendly	0	1	2	3
16. I enjoyed life	3	2	1	0

17. I had crying spells	0	1	2	3
18. I felt sad	0	1	2	3
19. I felt that people disliked me	0	1	2	3
20. I could not "get going"	0	1	2	3

Directions: Circle the number for each statement which best describes how often you felt or behaved this way *during the past week.*

Scoring: Add the numbers for each item you circled to get the total number of points.

Interpretation: While scoring lower than 16 is not a guarantee that you are not depressed, you are much less likely to suffer from clinical depression than if you score well above 16. If you scored higher than 16, you may be depressed, and you should seek help from a qualified professional—a psychologist or a psychiatrist or another physician. Among the treatments available for depression are various medications and psychotherapy.

shame to suffer needlessly. Depression is the most common psychiatric problem in the United States, and many instances go undiagnosed for years.

Days 5–7

Now that you are familiar with a wide variety of concepts important to changing eating-related behavior, it is worthwhile to engage in a period of careful self-observation. Self-observation (also called self-monitoring) is a good way to make yourself more aware of your current habits so you can focus your efforts in designing and carrying out your Personal Plan. As an added benefit, this period of self-observation will help you develop the habit of monitoring your behavior, both during the action phase of your Personal Plan and during the relapse-prevention phase (the rest of your life). It has been shown in research studies that successful long-term weight management is more likely among people who self-monitor than among those who do not.

How do you monitor your eating behavior? There are two aspects to the process: monitoring what you eat, and monitoring the circumstances of your eating. Chapter 6 will help you monitor what you eat, covering the basic nutritional information you need to become an educated "consumer." To monitor the circumstances of your eating is your task for the next three days. The Three-Day Eating Record (page 109) will help you do this.

Here's an example of a completed record for one day:

Day/Time	Type of Meal/Snack	Where Eaten	Circumstances
Monday			
8:30 A.M.	breakfast: coffee	kitchen	rushed
8:50 A.M.	snack: doughnut	car	passed store, looked good
noon	lunch: diet soda, candy bar	cafeteria	not hungry— no time, stressed
5:30 P.M.	snack: leftovers	out of refrigerator	very hungry
6 P.M.	dinner: pizza	den, in front of TV	tired, didn't want to cook

The idea is to eat in your usual manner. Do not try to eat "well" for the purposes of this exercise. Ideally, you will gain a better sense of the situations, time of day when you eat, and things that cause you to eat. You will also see the time pattern of your eating. As discussed, there are specific ways to change your eating habits for each situation if necessary.

What should you do with these monitoring forms? This depends on what you are most interested in monitoring. Once you have gained a better understanding of where your problem areas are, it is wise to focus on monitoring just one or two types of problem situations at a time. For example, you may decide to focus your monitoring on how you respond to stress at work, or how you deal with boredom. If so, your monitoring would focus on the times of day these are problems. You could keep track of exactly what you eat at those times and how well and often you substitute other activities for the inappropriate eating cues you are monitoring.

If you have a mathematical bent, you can even track frequencies of different behaviors. What percentage of stressful events leads you to overeat? Are you showing ongoing improvement? Are there new substitute behaviors you have thought of which can be added to your repertoire? By becoming a student of your own behavior, you will have the best chance of making permanent changes in your eating pattern and lifestyle. As you will see in the diet and exercise chapters, which follow, monitoring can be used to gain control in these areas, as well.

THREE-DAY EATING RECORD

Day/Time	Type of Meal/Snack	Where Eaten	Circumstances

Let's say you have learned, either from past experience or from this period of self-monitoring, that you need to stop eating when you are under stress at work but are not physically hungry. Eating is a habit that can briefly relieve stress and provide pleasure. Unfortunately, the relief is fleeting—and worse, it does nothing to address the source of the stress. In fact, it adds another stress in the form of a weight problem. How do you go about changing such a pattern of eating?

Many of my patients tell me that one of the greatest obstacles to stopping a habit like this is lack of awareness of the behavior while it is occurring. In other words, they say that they often don't realize they are eating as a stress reliever until it is too late—the snack has already been consumed. If there was a way to recognize the situation while there is still a chance to do something else instead of eating, the task of changing this and similar habits (such as eating out of boredom, or eating as a reward) would be much easier. I suggest a technique developed at the Johns Hopkins Weight Management Center which may work for you. It's called the "watch trick" and serves as a tap on the shoulder to help you to recognize inappropriate eating and to choose how you are going to respond.

Here's how to use it. If you are like most people, you wear a watch. (If not, buy or borrow one.) The beauty of a watch is that you tend to look at it periodically. In fact, you are likely to look at it at exactly those times when you are about to eat in response to inappropriate cues.

For example, you are bored. What time is it? How much longer until the show starts on television? Or, you are under stress at work—there's time pressure and an undesirable task to be done. Do I have to do it yet, or should I grab a snack first? What time is it?

Now we need a signal, a tap on the shoulder. Your watch is slightly annoying to you every time you lift your arm because *it is on upside down!* The 12 is on the bottom; the 6 is on the top. This is a gentle reminder to watch, not so much what you eat, but why you eat and whether your eating is being driven by bodily needs or by one of those inappropriate eating cues like stress or boredom.

Once alerted by the watch to the fact that you are considering eating, you can step back a moment and analyze the situation. First, are you physically hungry? If so, you are well justified in eating and should eat something. With your new awareness of your body's signals, you can eat without guilt because you will be eating appropriately, in response to your body's stated needs.

On the other hand, if you see your upside-down watch and remember that you recently ate or are not physically hungry, you are now aware that there is something else driving your urge to eat. Often you will be able to figure out what it is, or at least put it into one of the major categories of inappropriate eating cues described on Day 1 of the self-assessment in this chapter. If you can figure out what is causing you to want to eat when you are not hungry, you can now choose what to do about it.

The most appropriate response in most cases is to address the issue head-on. Stress? What can you do to address the source? Even writing down on a piece of paper, "I am stressed because of *X*" is a more effective stress reliever than temporarily avoiding the issue by eating. Better still, write down a plan to deal with the source of the stress. Boredom? As discussed, pick something to do from your lists of alternative activities. Do the same if you are using food as a reward.

With this tap on the shoulder, you have a choice. You can choose to go ahead and eat when you are not hungry, with all the lasting consequences it brings you (and such fleeting benefits). Or, you can recognize that you don't *need* to eat at this moment, and do something else. Urges to eat tend to last for only 10 or 15 minutes, so if you distract yourself briefly, the urge will usually pass.

Remember, you do not have to be perfect in your adherence to the plan described above. For example, if only half the times you were about to eat in response to an inappropriate cue you caught it in advance and responded appropriately, you will have a very important advantage in weight maintenance, now and after you have completed the action phase of your Personal Plan. This is because the difference between gaining weight and maintaining a stable weight is usually only 100 calories or less per day. Consistently cutting out an unneeded cookie or two a day is the difference between weight gain and stable weight.

One other factor is worth emphasizing. In some ways, it gets easier to avoid inappropriate eating the more experienced you become at monitoring yourself, using either the "watch trick" or other means, such as keeping food records. This is because appropriate eating and appropriate responses to stress, boredom, and the like are learned habits. Respond appropriately to a stressful situation a few times in a row instead of eating, and you will find that this is a far more satisfying response than eating. You will find that you are in much better control, not only of your eating, but of your stress, as well. This is a reward that eating cannot provide, and this reward will make it increasingly easy to respond appropriately.

Putting Your Assessment to Work

You have now performed a thorough self-assessment of your eating-related behaviors, and you have learned a few techniques to change the inappropriate ones. If you have completed the assessment faithfully and honestly, you have learned some things about your eating habits that will help you lose weight and, more importantly, keep it off for the long haul.

To put this information to good use, you will now learn how to incorporate the behavioral assessment and change techniques into the action and maintenance phases of your Personal Plan.

There are five areas we must review in formulating the critical behavioral portion of your Personal Plan. They are listed in order of priority.

1. Review your assessments for depression and binge-eating disorders and seek help if there is a problem.
2. Review your motivations for losing weight (Chapter 2) and explore the significance of food in your life. Rededicate yourself to your Personal Plan of Action.
3. Develop and write down a repertoire of flexible responses to use when faced with inappropriate eating cues to which you are susceptible.
4. Begin monitoring your eating-related behavior. Make monitoring a permanent part of your Personal Plan. Use the "watch trick" and substitute appropriate responses for eating in response to inappropriate eating cues.
5. Begin following the advice you find useful in controlling your eating.

Your Personal Plan can include a collection of miscellaneous behavioral tools which can help you gain control of your eating. Not all of them will work for everyone all of the time, but all of them can be helpful in the right setting. Pick a few that make sense to you from the following descriptions, and write them down as part of your Personal Plan.

1. Use smaller plates for meals. They hold less and look fuller with less food.
2. Serve yourself a reasonable portion of food for each meal and forbid seconds. Help yourself stick to this by cleaning up the kitchen and putting away serving dishes *before* you start eating. Serving dishes left out on the table, counter, or stove are a source of temptation.
3. If you are still hungry after a reasonably-sized meal, have a noncaloric cold or hot drink or a piece of fruit or sugar-free gum. Get busy at once doing something non–food related. If you are still hungry later, have another noncaloric drink, stick of gum, or piece of fruit.
4. Slow down your eating pace to allow the satiety signal to get through. Chew your food completely (this also aids digestion). Put down your eating utensil between each bite of the meal.
5. Limit where you eat to one room of your home—preferably the kitchen or dining room.

6. Do not allow eating in front of the television. Do not do other things while eating. Concentrate on the eating.
7. Enjoy much smaller but more frequent servings of the foods you like. A sliver of chocolate cake, consumed slowly and in small bites, savoring it as it melts in your mouth, will give you better "value" for your calories.
8. Buy only single serving sizes, not economy sizes, of foods that you have trouble controlling your intake of.
9. Brush your teeth immediately after eating. This may inhibit you from snacking soon after the meal (particularly dinner).

Finally, integrate the behavior change aspects of your Personal Plan with the diet and exercise aspects. To do this, it is vital that you recognize that behavior change is the essence of changing your diet and becoming more physically fit. If you temporarily restrict your diet and engage in lots of exercise in order to lose weight, but you do not make permanent changes in the kinds of food you eat, portion sizes, and the amount of physical activity you get, the weight loss will be only temporary. In order to maintain weight loss, you need to make permanent changes in three areas of your lifestyle: behavior, nutrition, and activity level.

As you read the next two chapters, keep in mind that your aim is to make behavior changes you can stick with, without deprivation, for the rest of your life. This can be done if you use the tools you learned in this chapter.

Now turn the page and begin planning a personal diet that you will be happy to make a part of your Personal Plan of Action.

SIX

What's a "Good" Diet, Anyway?

In the early part of this century, our understanding of what humans need in the way of nutrients was very limited compared to what it is today. At that time, many Americans were faced with food shortages and nutrient imbalances, which created widespread hunger and malnutrition. When it became obvious that our national interest would be better served by a population of well-fed and healthy workers who were full of energy, many groups in government, academia, and industry worked diligently to develop more healthful foods, and to distribute them efficiently to all segments of the population. For example, crops and animals have been genetically modified so that they are more nutritious and produce more edible products; consider, too, that foods are safer and more widely available because of new methods of preservation and rapid transportation; finally, the government now carefully monitors food handling, packaging, and labeling to safeguard the health of consumers. A significant part of this focus on developing a nutritious, plentiful, and safe food supply has been the establishment of nationally approved guidelines for good eating.

Surrounded by a vast amount of food offering plenty of nutrients, however, many of us still make unwise food choices. We often eat a diet that is too low in some critical nutrients and too high in others. For example, many women routinely consume less than the Recommended Dietary Allowances (RDA) for calcium, iron, vitamins A and C, and fiber, and yet many of those same women appear *over*nourished because of excess caloric intake and the resulting excess body fat. Eating too many calories also tends to result in taking in more sodium, sugar, alcohol, cholesterol, and saturated fat than is healthy. So, while plenty is available to all, all are not choosing well.

Our most obvious imbalance is excess dietary energy—too many calories. Because our food is abundant and energy rich, we find ourselves caught in an evolutionary paradox. On the one hand, evolution has built into us an intense biological drive to consume everything available, to "store up" in anticipation of a time when food isn't plentiful. On the other hand, we have developed skills and technologies that release us from the need to spend much energy in the pursuit of our food, so that not many of us farm or hunt for our food. For most of us, energy intake (eating foods) and energy expenditure (the pursuit of finding food to eat) have become uncoupled. The problem of hunger for too many Americans has been replaced with the problem of "never being hungry." We are in a state of calorie overload.

In this land of plenty, what is a "good" diet, anyway? Obviously, it is important to eat enough nutritious food to prevent illness and disease. However, it is equally important to carefully select what we eat in order to balance high nutrient needs with appropriate calorie intake.

Dietary Guidelines and the Food Guide Pyramid

The Overview

The most current "good diet" recommendations are the Dietary Guidelines for Americans published in 1995, which reflect federal nutrition policy distilled from a wealth of scientific information. These guidelines promote greater intake of some nutrients and discourage overconsumption of others. The guidelines are:

1. Eat a variety of foods.
2. Balance the food you eat with physical activity. Maintain or improve your weight.
3. Choose a diet with plenty of grain products, vegetables, and fruits.
4. Choose a diet low in fat, saturated fat, and cholesterol.
5. Choose a diet moderate in sugar.
6. Choose a diet moderate in salt and sodium.
7. If you drink alcoholic beverages, do so in moderation.

Though simply stated, these directives when put together form a complete picture of self-managed, lifelong eating for good health. By following guidelines 1 and 3 you can ensure that your diet contains enough of all the nutrients to help prevent deficiency diseases and perhaps even some chronic illnesses. Guidelines 4, 5, 6, and 7 specifically caution against overconsuming various food substances that are known to increase the risk of heart disease, stroke, cancer, diabetes, high blood pressure, and liver disease. Finally, guideline 2 can be met by combining all the other guidelines with appropriate physical activity.

These, then, are the guidelines for a good diet that have been established by the federal government after exhaustive study of the energy and nutrition needs of the human body. By following these guidelines, the person who is at a reasonable weight can maintain that weight and increase his or her chances of avoiding many illnesses. Once calorie imbalance has resulted in obesity, however, a weight-reducing plan of some kind is needed.

A Closer Look

In 1992 the U.S. Department of Agriculture, along with the Department of Health and Human Services, devised a visual representation of guidelines 1-5, which naturally fell into a pyramid shape. The aptly named Food Guide Pyramid (page 118) is composed of five major (nutrient-dense) food groups, capped off by a sixth category representing foods that are low in nutrients but high in calories. The energy in the sixth group comes mostly from fat, simple sugars, or both. (In other words, the sixth category provides mostly "empty calories"— calories with relatively little nutritional value.) By choosing from the five major groups, you are most likely to eat a *variety* of foods for basic nutrient adequacy. Simply by choosing to eat more *vegetables, fruits,* and *grains,* and limiting extra *sugars* and *fats,* you can increase the likelihood of *maintaining* or *improving* your weight.

The last two dietary guidelines (6 and 7) recommend minimizing the use of both sodium and alcohol. They are not depicted in the Food Guide Pyramid, but they are taken into account when developing a good diet, particularly for weight management.

Sodium is an element of sodium chloride, also known as salt. Sodium has important functions in the body. People can easily consume adequate amounts of salt just by choosing the recommended number of foods from the five major groups, and they can easily *overdo* the salt in an unhealthy way by adding it to foods either in cooking or at the table. To avoid consuming too much salt, temper your temptation to season with salt from the shaker, and avoid eating (or at least limit) the following foods, which contain excess sodium: cured and pickled foods, highly processed and salted snacks, many canned vegetables and soups, cheeses, and soy sauce and other condiments.

For people who retain excess amounts of water or who have high blood pressure, it is especially important to control sodium intake. Most health authorities agree that 3,000 milligrams, or 3 grams, of

PUTTING THE DIETARY GUIDELINES INTO ACTION: THE FOOD GUIDE PYRAMID

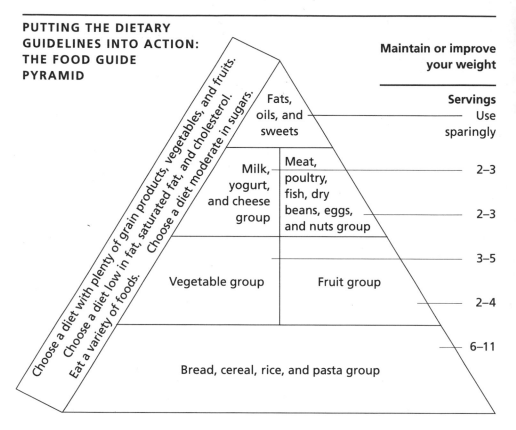

sodium per day is not harmful for most people. Keep in mind that 3 grams is only about one-tenth of an ounce! It's important to keep in mind, too, that while it is very easy to consume too much sodium, sodium *does not* contribute energy or calories to the diet and does not cause a person to gain fat weight. Controlling sodium intake may help you to control how much water you retain (bloating) or help you to control high blood pressure (an important enough reason), but it will not help you to lose excess body fat. In fact, reducing salt *too much* can interfere with your weight reduction success: if you restrict salt to the point where your food doesn't taste very good, that may make it harder for you to stick to a weight reduction food plan. Of course, creative use of other flavorings and spices can make low-salt foods much more appealing.

Alcohol consumption is a different matter. Eliminating or cutting back on alcohol *can* help you to control overall calories, and therefore body weight. Alcoholic beverages contain very few if any necessary nutrients, but many calories—many *empty* calories. Each gram of alcohol has 7 calories. This is more than sugar, at 4 calories per gram, and nearly as much as fat, at 9 calories per gram. Also, in mixed drinks, the beverage combined with the alcohol (such as soda, cream, or fruit juice) often contributes hundreds of extra empty calories, either as carbohydrates or as fats. Only in the case of fruit juice are key nutrients contributed.

There's a "one-two punch" that often goes along with the consumption of alcoholic beverages—alcohol is most often consumed in a social setting, where high-calorie snack foods or large meals are readily available. Since alcohol lowers defenses (causing disinhibition—a state of no longer being inhibited or restrained), many people eat more of this food than they would under ordinary circumstances. To complicate matters, it seems that the body may slow down its fat-burning processes when alcohol is present. The body seems to prefer to burn alcohol before fat, perhaps in an effort to rid itself of this toxin. While the body is busily burning the alcohol, it's storing away the fat.

A Closer Look at Dietary Guideline 2

For many Americans, the most elusive dietary guideline is "Maintain or improve your weight." Many feel confident that they have already cut back on total fat, reduced sodium intake, limited alcoholic beverages, and significantly cut down on cholesterol. What they may not realize, however, is that they probably haven't reduced the total calories consumed; in fact, for most Americans, average caloric intake has *increased* slightly in the past decade.

The upswing in caloric intake is partly due to a failure to control the size of portions or servings of food. Most restaurants, for example, specialize in serving larger than necessary amounts—and Americans eat out *a lot*. Also, although many people have learned to budget their fat intake, they have often neglected to recognize that eating unlimited amounts of fat-free foods (which, it's worth noting, are not *calorie free*) will make them gain weight. Understanding what counts as a serving is a key issue for all foods and will be explained in more detail later in this chapter (in the discussion of the three-day dietary evaluation). In addition to overeating, many people are less active than ever, and so the average American's body weight and body fat have been steadily increasing.

According to the latest government surveys, at least one-third of American adults are now overweight. (Overweight is defined as being at least 20 percent heavier than ideal body weight, or IBW.) To deter-

TABLE 6.1 HEALTHY WEIGHT RANGES FOR MEN AND WOMEN

Height without Shoes	Weight in Pounds without Clothes	Height without Shoes	Weight in Pounds without Clothes
5'0"	97–128	5'10"	132–174
5'1"	101–132	5'11"	136–179
5'2"	104–137	6'0"	140–184
5'3"	107–141	6'1"	144–189
5'4"	111–146	6'2"	148–195
5'5"	114–150	6'3"	152–200
5'6"	118–155	6'4"	156–205
5'7"	121–160	6'5"	160–211
5'8"	125–164	6'6"	164–216
5'9"	129–169		

Note: The higher weights in the ranges generally apply to men, who tend to have more muscle and bone; the lower weights more often apply to women, who have less muscle and bone.

Source: Derived from National Research Council, *Recommended Dietary Allowances*, 10th ed. (Washington, D.C.: National Research Council, National Academy of Sciences, 1989).

mine where your current weight falls on the IBW scale, consult table 6.1, "Healthy Weight Ranges for Men and Women." If you are over your IBW, you can find out what percentage you're over by subtracting your IBW from your current weight and then dividing that number by your IBW.

For example, suppose you weigh 200 pounds. The highest IBW in your height and weight category is 160 pounds; subtracting 160 pounds from 200 pounds, you get a difference of 40 pounds. Divide 40 pounds by 160 pounds, and you'll find that you are 25 percent over your highest IBW: 200 − 160 = 40; 40 ÷ 160 = 0.25, or 25 percent.

If your weight currently falls within your designated range for ideal body weight, congratulations! We encourage you to make every effort to maintain this weight by balancing your food intake with appropriate physical activity. On the other hand, if you are 20 percent or more above IBW, you are considered overweight and may be at increased risk of developing high blood pressure, diabetes, and high blood cholesterol levels.

While most experts use ideal body weight to assess relative health risks and establish treatment guidelines, many do not point to the

IBW as the optimum weight goal for a particular individual. This is partly because body weight includes more than just fat; it also reflects bone frame and density, internal organs, and muscle mass. Therefore, IBW may be 120 pounds for one woman who is 5'2" tall, but 108 pounds may be best for another woman who is the same height but who has a smaller frame or is less muscular.

It is also apparent from many research studies that some degree of excess body fat may not impose significant health risks. Consequently, a rather broad range of weight, from 10 percent below IBW to 20 percent above IBW, is considered to be reasonably healthy for most people. (To determine a weight that is 20 percent above IBW, multiply the highest IBW in your height and weight category by 1.20; for example, 20 percent over the highest ideal body weight for a person who is 5'11" tall is 194 × 1.20 = 232 pounds. To determine a weight that is 10 percent below IBW, multiply the lowest IBW in your category by .90: 151 x .90 = 135 pounds.) For some people, even weights of more than 20 percent over IBW may not be unduly harmful, because of individual genetic and lifestyle factors. On the other hand, even a small amount of excess body weight may be medically risky if it is distributed around the abdomen, as discussed in Chapter 1.

Recent studies have shown that many seriously overweight people can substantially reduce their health risks by losing only 10 percent of their total body weight. For example, a woman who weighs 200 pounds but who ideally should weigh 120 pounds may be able to control her diabetes by reducing her weight to 180 pounds and maintaining more healthful eating habits. For her, "improving" her weight may be very beneficial, even though she will still be approximately 60 pounds over the ideal.

Using the Food Guide Pyramid for Good Health and Good Weight

By following the general principles of the Food Guide Pyramid, you can achieve healthful eating habits and ensure good nutrition. You can eat enough and avoid eating too much.

Let's look at the five major food groups more closely. All of the foods within a major food group have one or more key nutrients in common. The bread, cereal, rice, and pasta group, for example, provides energy in the form of complex carbohydrates and is a good source of B vitamins, minerals, and fiber. The foods in the vegetable group are generally low in calories, provide energy mostly from complex carbohydrates, and are good sources of vitamins A and C, folic acid, magnesium, iron, and fiber. Fruits contribute Vitamin C, Vitamin A, potassium, and fiber to the diet. They are also relatively low in calories and provide energy from simple and complex carbohydrates. These three groups compose the lower two levels of the pyramid. Most of these foods are low in fats and added sugars but are bulky with water and fiber. They are all derived from plants.

The milk, yogurt, and cheese group and the meat, poultry, fish, dry beans, eggs, and nuts group are derived mostly from animal sources. They provide high levels of protein, iron, zinc, and calcium as well as vitamins D and B-12. But many of these foods also contribute high levels of fat, including artery-clogging saturated fat and cholesterol. Therefore, while some milk and meat or meat substitute foods are desirable in the diet to meet overall nutritional needs, you should not eat too much of them. A person who eats too much of these foods is likely to take in way more protein than is needed. Protein, especially from animal sources, can be a costly source of calories. Excess protein can also overburden the liver and kidneys, which must process protein; it may also contribute to the development of osteoporosis, because excess protein intake makes the body excrete too much calcium in the urine.

By choosing foods from the five major groups in the recommended proportions, most people will eat more vegetables, fruits, and grains, and limit extra sugars and fats. The structure of the pyramid illustrates the nutritional concepts of *proportionality, variety,* and *moderation,* all of which contribute to overall dietary *balance.*

The order in which the five major groups are stacked, and their relative positions in the pyramid outline, illustrate dietary *proportionality.* It is obvious from the large amount of space in the pyramid dedicated to the bread, cereals, rice, and pasta group—the grains—that these foods should figure most prominently in our diets. They serve as the foundation of a good diet. Fruits and vegetables compose the next level up from the foundation. They are lined up side by side to reflect their similar botanical origins and the overlap of some of their key nutrients. Again, the amount of space dedicated to fruits and vegetables means that we should consume lots of the foods in these groups.

As we approach the top of the pyramid, where it narrows, we see that space is allocated for smaller amounts of iron-rich and calcium-rich protein foods. These are primarily of animal origin, such as meats, poultry, fish, and dairy products, but include a few plant foods, as well, such as beans, nuts, and seeds. The tip of the pyramid depicts the negligible role that low-nutrient but high-calorie foods should play in our overall food plans. These empty-calorie foods provide energy with very few nutrients.

For each of the five major food groups, there is a recommended range of servings which corresponds to the amount of space each food group is allocated within the pyramid. Eating at least the minimum number of servings from each group, using a *variety* of specific food choices, helps ensure healthful levels of all the key nutrients. A nutritious, three-meal-a-day pattern of servings might look like this:

Breakfast	Lunch	Dinner
3 bread	3 bread	3 bread
2 fruit/vegetable	2 fruit/vegetable	2 fruit/vegetable
1 milk	1 milk	1 milk
1 meat	1 meat	1 meat

By varying the number of servings within the recommended range, total calories for the day can be manipulated to meet individual needs (this is what is meant by *moderation*). For example, rather than consuming a total of nine servings from the bread and cereal group, reducing the number of servings of bread at each meal to two, for total daily consumption of six servings (still within the recommended guidelines, but at the lower end) can result in moderate weight loss.

Total calories can also be manipulated by choosing either high-fat or low-fat food items from each group. By choosing the foods lowest in fat from each of the five groups and limiting servings to the minimum number recommended, a woman wanting to lose weight could reduce calories to between 1200 and 1400 per day. Conversely, an active teenage boy choosing at the high end of the serving ranges and not limiting his choices based on fat content, with a few extras from the pyramid tip (fats, oils, and sweets), could consume as many as 3000 calories—and not gain weight.

It's easy to see how useful the pyramid is as a guide for a wide range of healthy people who are choosing a *balanced* diet. All the nutrients are provided in adequate, but not excessive, amounts for maintaining good health while simultaneously balancing energy intake with energy needs to maintain or improve body weight.

Remember, you can follow the general guidelines provided by the pyramid, but you also need to tailor them to fit your own specific needs, especially if your goal is to lose weight yet maintain a nutritious diet. For most people, weight loss or preventing weight gain can be achieved by manipulating food choices to stay within certain calorie limits. A big part of the equation, of course, is physical activity: the number of calories that you can consume and still maintain or lower your weight is determined to a great extent by the amount and kind of physical activity you do. The trick is to set goals and choose a plan based on *your* individual nutrient and energy needs. Later in this chapter we'll explain how to determine your individual nutrient and energy needs, evaluate your current diet, and choose your own personal strategies for weight reduction. Before getting to that, however, we need to take a look at calorie balance and fat.

Calories Still Count

Everyone burns energy, every day. We measure this energy in calories. Food provides us with fuel (measured in calories) to burn for our energy needs and with structural components for our bodies, plus other nutrients (vitamins and minerals) to aid in these two processes. When the energy you eat equals the energy you burn, then your weight remains stable. The equation looks like this:

Calories (in) = Calories (out) = stable weight

On the other hand, when energy eaten exceeds energy burned, then weight is gained:

Calories (in) > Calories (out) = weight gain

Of course, when energy eaten is less than daily energy burned, then extra calories stored in the body as fat are burned up, and weight is lost:

Calories (in) < Calories (out) = weight loss

If you need to lose weight, most authorities agree that gradual weight loss is better for you than rapid loss. Gradual loss is usually defined as between half a pound and two pounds per week. If you are a small woman, you can expect to lose half a pound to one pound per week when you follow a well-balanced, low-calorie food plan. If you are a woman with a medium to large structure, you are likely to lose one to two pounds per week. Men's energy needs are often higher than women's. For that reason, men tend to lose weight more rapidly, commonly two to three pounds per week.

When people lose weight at higher rates than these, it may mean that their food plan is not providing enough nutrition for their energy needs. It is difficult for anyone to obtain the minimum nutrient requirements when consuming fewer than 1200 calories per day. In other words, fewer than 1200 calories per day can promote faster loss than one half to two pounds per week, but often at the expense of muscle mass, good nutrition, and general well-being. Rapid weight loss should not be undertaken except under medical supervision with specialized nutritional supplements.

Gradual weight loss usually reflects a thoughtful, careful refining of food habits rather than a "crash diet." The diet you are designing for your Personal Plan of Action is a "normal," more natural and healthful diet. If it is practiced long enough to promote significant weight loss, it can become a permanent lifestyle change.

A carefully constructed food plan for healthful eating and gradual weight loss can be your blueprint for successful weight maintenance, as well. For example, if you currently eat at the high end of the pyramid ranges for the five food groups plus an average of six servings daily from the fats, oils, and sweets, then you may be able to narrow your pyramid by eating fewer servings from the five major groups and eliminating or reducing choices from the tip. After weight loss is complete, you may be able to increase your calories slightly for maintenance. You can do this by following the pyramid guidelines while increasing the total number of servings to a level in between your old food habits and the level you use for weight loss.

Where should you increase servings when you move from the weight loss to the weight maintenance pyramid? It is best to use the plant-based food groups: grains, fruits, and vegetables. This allows you to increase the amount of food you eat with only a moderate increase in calories. The reason is that these food groups almost entirely contain low-fat or fat-free foods. Fat, which is found mostly in the other three food groups, is the most *fattening* of the three macronutrients (protein, carbohydrate, and fat), even though it takes up the smallest space both in your foods and in the pyramid.

Why Is Fat Fattening?

There are at least four reasons why high-fat foods trigger the consumption of too many calories and promote weight gain.

1. Fat provides more than twice as many calories as an equal amount of protein or carbohydrate.
2. Fat contributes very appealing flavors and textures to food, which promotes overeating.
3. The more fat present in a meal, the less some of us are able to balance daily intake against daily energy needs.
4. When too many total calories are eaten, carbohydrate is burned preferentially while fat tends to be efficiently stored, particularly when you are inactive.

Let's examine each of these points more carefully.

Fats of both animal and plant origin are very dense sources of calories. Every kind of fat, including olive oil, butter, beef fat, lard, coconut oil, and corn oil, whether liquid or solid, has approximately 9 to 10 calories per gram. Compare this with carbohydrates, which have only 4 calories per gram. Protein, too, has only 4 calories per gram. This means that a lot of fat calories can fit in a small package. For example, a medium-sized baked potato has 150 to 200 calories, but the much smaller 2 tablespoons of margarine that go on top more than doubles the calories—and every single one of those margarine calories comes from fat.

Another way to look at this principle is to envision two glasses of milk, one whole milk, one skim, each exactly 8 fluid ounces. The whole milk contains 10 grams of fat and has about 170 calories, but the skim milk is nearly fat-free and has only about 90 calories. The amount of milk is the same, one cup, but the removal of the butterfat from the whole milk cuts the calories in half for the skim milk.

Many food components contribute flavor to our foods, including salt, sugar, acids, herbs, and spices, but the addition of fat in combination with these components is especially appealing to most of us. Fats often have flavors of their own which tend to carry through or boost other flavors. Fats also impart desirable textures to foods such as tenderness in baked products, crispiness in fried foods, moistness or juiciness in meats, and smoothness in candies and frozen desserts. Fatty foods are the most likely to be overeaten, often beyond the point of fullness, and can make you want to eat even when you're not hungry. Think about how many times your stomach has growled when you smelled sizzling bacon, or how often you eat a rich dessert even when you "don't have room for it." Many foods that are high in fat content, particularly those that are combined with sugar or salt, or both, are often eaten for fun or comfort rather than for need.

High-fat foods are not only dangerously appealing to our senses, but recent evidence indicates that high-fat meals seem to be less filling than high-carbohydrate meals. In other words, we don't feel as full during or right after a high-fat meal as we do when the meal is high in carbohydrates, or we may feel equally full despite a large difference in total calories. This combination of sensory appeal and delayed or reduced fullness can result in eating too many calories without realizing it. For some people, eating a high-fat, high-calorie meal doesn't suppress the amount of food they consume at the next meal. Since automatic adjustments in food consumption may not occur during the high-fat meal itself, and the high-fat meal may not be compensated for later, total calories for the day will often be higher than needed.

When too many calories are eaten, but the calories come from carbohydrate rather than fat, the body tends to burn off some or all of the extra calories through a slight increase in metabolism. Conversely, extra calories from fat *do not* promote an increase in metabolism and are very quickly and efficiently stored as body fat; 97 calories of an extra 100 calories consumed as fat *will be stored*. When extra calories come from both carbohydrate and fat, most of the carbohydrate calories are used first, either right away or sometime later, between meals, because they are easily removed from temporary storage in the liver and because we may be inefficient at converting them into fat. However, extra fat is automatically transported into semi-permanent fat storage and is only burned during prolonged physical exertion or after carbohydrate stores are depleted—in other words, when you go on a calorie-deficient diet.

In summary, fat is fattening because it tastes so good that we tend to eat more than we need. It has more than twice as many calories per unit weight as other food sources, and our bodies prefer to store fat rather than to burn it, particularly when we are inactive or excess calories are present—or both.

By switching to a lower fat way of eating we can eat just as much as, and sometimes a little more than, we usually do, and avoid progressive weight gain. For most people, lowering overall fat intake automatically promotes the selection of more healthful foods. For some people, the result is a substantial decrease in total calories and, thus, weight loss. Using fat-budgeting (which means limiting fat calories to between 15 and 25 percent of the total caloric intake) along with a high-nutrient, portion-controlled food plan and physical activity, most people will achieve gradual but significant weight loss with a minimum of deprivation.

Here's the lowdown on fat and calories, and how you can reduce your intake of both:

1. **Avoid using fat as flavoring in cooking or at the table.**
   Avoid rich sauces on vegetables and potatoes.
   Eat bread without butter or margarine.
   Reduce butter, margarine, and oil in recipes.
   Eat potatoes without butter or margarine.
   Eat vegetables without butter or margarine.
   Bake, broil, or poach fish and shellfish rather than fry them.
2. **Limit high-fat meats and meat substitutes (eat one or two vegetarian meals per day).**
   Use vegetarian tomato sauce on pasta.
   Limit hamburger, most lunch meats, and hot dogs.
   Eat small (2–4 oz.) servings of lean meat at any one time.
   Eat beef, pork, and lamb infrequently.
   Eat small amounts of chicken, fish, and beans more often.
   Eat low-fat cheese or vegetarian pizza.
   Avoid excessive use of whole eggs, nuts, and seeds.
3. **Modify your choices.**
   Purchase low-fat or fat-free versions of your favorite crackers and chips.
   Buy low-fat or fat-free cheese (less than 6 grams of fat per ounce).
   Remove skin from chicken and remove visible fat from meat.
   Use skim or 1 percent milk rather than whole or 2 percent.
   Eat fat-free frozen yogurt instead of regular ice cream.
   Replace cream or whole milk in recipes with evaporated skim milk.
4. **Use specially manufactured fat-free or low-fat food substitutes.**
   Use cooking spray in baking pans or skillets.
   Use lemon juice, vinegar, or nonfat dressing on salad.
   Use fat-free mayonnaise instead of regular.
   Use low-fat or fat-free plain yogurt instead of sour cream.
   Use fat-free cream cheese on bagels and in recipes.
   Use light or whipped margarine, or fat-free substitutes, instead of butter or regular margarine.
   Replace whole eggs with egg substitutes.
5. **Replace one food choice with another.**
   Spread jelly, jam, or apple butter on toast or bread instead of butter or margarine.

Eat fruit for dessert or a snack instead of cakes, candy bars, cookies, or ice cream.

Eat pretzels instead of potato chips.

Suck on hard candy or chew gum instead of eating a chocolate candy bar.

Replace high-fat breakfast meats (bacon, sausage) with Canadian bacon.

Pulling It All Together for Your Personal Plan of Action

So far in this chapter we have looked closely at three important dietary elements for healthy weight loss and maintenance: *choosing foods according to the pyramid guidelines* to optimize health and well-being; modestly *reducing total calories* to create a negative energy balance for gradual weight loss (with an eventual increase to a neutral balance for maintenance); and *limiting total fat* to further promote burning of stored fat and to increase the volume of food you can eat while staying within your calorie budget.

Now it's time to put these three dietary elements together into your Personal Plan of Action. To begin, use the following worksheet, proceeding through the eight steps to decide (1) what your personal goal weight is and (2) how many calories, fat grams, and pyramid servings you should eat daily to achieve a gradual loss of 0.5 to 2.0 pounds per week.

WORKSHEET FOR ESTABLISHING GOALS AND DIETARY BUDGETS

Step 1.

Record your current weight (in pounds), height (in inches), sex, and age:

Weight: _____ Height: _____ Sex: _____ Age: _____

Step 2.

Using tables 6.2 through 6.5, determine the number of calories you are probably eating now to maintain your current weight.

First, use table 6.2 to find your Body Surface Area. With your left index finger locate your weight (to the nearest 10 pounds) in the left-hand column of the table. Then find your height (to the nearest inch) across the top of the table with your right index finger. By moving your left finger across and your right finger down, find the number where your fingers meet. This number is your Body Surface Area (BSA). Record it here.

My BSA is: _____.

Second, choose either table 6.3 or 6.4, depending upon whether you are female or male. With your left index finger, locate your age (to the nearest whole number, rounding up) in the left-hand column. With your right index finger, locate your BSA (from table 6.2) along the top of the table. Move your left finger across and your right finger down until they meet. This number is a close approximation of the number of calories you are presently burning in 24 hours *at rest,* and is called your Resting Metabolic Rate (RMR). Record it here.

My RMR is: _____.

Now, use table 6.5 to determine your *total daily energy needs.* This is the number of calories you probably are eating each day to *maintain* your *current* weight. In table 6.5, use your left index finger to find the closest value corresponding to your RMR (from table 6.3 or table 6.4) in the left-hand column (when in doubt, round down). With your right index finger, choose an activity factor which reflects your *average* activity level, according to the following descriptions:

1.3 = Inactive.
Sitting at a desk all day, watching TV or reading all evening. No fidgeting.

1.5 = Active.
Sporadic movement throughout the day, such as doing light household chores, walking up and down numerous flights of stairs while working. (Most people fall into this category.)

1.7 = Very Active.
Daily strenuous workouts, heavy housework, frequently engaging in physical sports.

Moving your fingers across and down, find your predicted total daily energy needs and record that figure here.

My total daily energy needs are: _____.

You will refer back to this number when you get to Step 5.

Step 3.
According to your height, find your *Reasonable, Healthy Weight (RHW) range* in table 6.1, "Healthy Weight Ranges for Men and Women." If you are a man, your RHW is toward the higher end of the range. If you are a woman, your RHW is in the lower end of the range.

My RHW range is between _____ and _____ pounds.

Next, choose a comfortable realistic goal weight in your RHW range.

I am comfortable with a goal weight of _____ pounds.

And subtract your goal weight from your current weight.

The difference between my current weight and my goal weight is _____ pounds.

If this amount of weight seems too overwhelming to tackle, then start with a weight loss goal of losing 10 percent of your current weight. (Multiply your present weight by .90 to find your goal weight, or multiply your present weight by .10 to find out how many pounds you are planning to lose. For example, suppose you weigh 200 pounds and you want to lose 10 percent of your current weight. Multiply $200 \times .90 = 180$ pounds, which is your personal goal weight. Or, $200 \times .10 = 20$ pounds that you are planning to lose.) After you have lost the initial 10 percent, you can decide whether to continue losing weight. If you wish to lose further, you can do so in 5-pound or 10-pound increments until you are satisfied. In no case, though, should you reduce to below the lower end of the RHW range for your height and age.

My current weight is _____ pounds $\times .90 =$ initial goal weight of _____ pounds. This is a difference of _____ pounds from my current weight.

Step 4.
Choosing from the options that you calculated in Step 3, you have decided that you would like to lose _____ pounds. To determine the amount of time it will take to lose this weight at various rates of weight loss per week, multiply the number of pounds you wish to lose (either ultimately or initially) by all the factors below.

A. Number of pounds _____ $\times 2.0 =$ _____ weeks to lose an average of *0.5 pounds per week*. (This is the preferred rate of loss if you have fewer than 10 pounds to lose.)

B. Number of pounds _____ $\times 1.0 =$ _____ weeks to lose an average of *1 pound per week*.

C. Number of pounds _____ $\times 0.67 =$ _____ weeks to lose an average of *1.5 pounds per week*.

D. Number of pounds _____ × 0.5 = _____ weeks to lose an average of *2 pounds per week.*

Step 5.

Complete the appropriate equation below to decide on your daily weight loss calorie budget based on how much you would like to lose per week (see Step 4).

My current daily energy needs (from Step 2 and table 6.5) are: _____ calories per day. This figure minus:

A. 250 calories = _____ *calories/day for 0.5 pounds per week loss.* (Again, this is the preferred rate of loss if you have fewer than 10 pounds to lose.)

B. 500 calories = _____ *calories/day for 1.0 pounds per week loss.*

C. 750 calories = _____ *calories/day for 1.5 pounds per week loss.*

D. 1,000 calories = _____ *calories/day for 2.0 pounds per week loss.*

E. 1,500 calories = _____ *calories/day for 3.0 pounds per week loss.* (This rate of weight loss is to be considered only if you have more than 100 pounds to lose, and then must be done only under the supervision of a physician.)

Now, record what your daily calorie intake is going to be:

I have chosen my weight loss calorie level to be _____ calories per day in order to lose _____ pounds per week.

Ask yourself whether this level of daily calories seems realistic. Keep in mind that the faster you lose, the less time it will take but the stricter you must be. The tendency is to try to lose as quickly as possible, but many people find that the caloric sacrifice is too high a price to pay. You may want to work your daily calorie level down gradually until you reach the lowest level that is comfortable for you. As discussed in chapters 2 and 5, excessive deprivation often makes it less likely that you will be able to succeed in staying on target in your Personal Plan. It is important not to choose a rate of loss that results in a calorie level below 1200 for a woman or 1500 for a man, since below these levels it can be difficult to take in enough vitamins and minerals. If the equation you chose above indicates a required calorie level below 1200 calories, then start with 1200 calories per day. This will balance your nutritional health with your desired rate of loss. If you are unable to lose weight on 1200 calories per day, you may have a metabolic condition such as hypothyroidism and should seek the advice of a physician or a physician-directed weight loss center.

Step 6.
Based on the calorie level for weight loss which you chose in Step 5, choose a calorie range and corresponding pyramid pattern from the choices in table 6.6. Find the column corresponding to your total daily calorie range across the top, then look down the column to see how many servings of each of the food groups you should eat daily. These patterns were calculated based on your choosing the lowest fat, lowest calorie foods in each of the five major food groups.

I have chosen my calorie range to be between _____ and _____ calories. My pyramid pattern calls for the following number of servings in each of the food groups:

bread:____ vegetable:____ fruit:____ milk:____

meat:____ fats, oils, sweets:____

Step 7.
Based on the range of calories you plan to eat per day as determined in Step 6, choose a daily *fat gram budget* from table 6.7. These fat budgets account for 15 to 25 percent of total calories.

My daily fat budget is ____ to ____ grams.

Step 8.
Now it's time to summarize your goals and dietary budgets.

I currently weigh ____ pounds.

My personal goal weight is ____ pounds.

My goal is to lose ____ pounds in ____ weeks,
by losing about ____ pounds per week.

To achieve my goal I will eat:

—within my budget of ____ to ____ calories per day.

—according to the following pyramid pattern:
____ servings of bread, ____ servings of vegetables, ____ servings of fruit, ____ servings of milk, ____ servings of meat, and ____ servings of fats/oils/sweets.

—within my budget of ____ to ____ grams of fat per day.

TABLE 6.2 BODY SURFACE AREA

Weight (Lbs)	Height (Inches)						
	60	61	62	63	64	65	66
100	1.4	1.4	1.4	1.4	1.5	1.5	1.5
110	1.4	1.5	1.5	1.5	1.5	1.5	1.6
120	1.5	1.5	1.5	1.6	1.6	1.6	1.6
130	1.6	1.6	1.6	1.6	1.6	1.6	1.7
140	1.6	1.6	1.6	1.7	1.7	1.7	1.7
150	1.7	1.7	1.7	1.7	1.7	1.8	1.8
160	1.7	1.7	1.7	1.8	1.8	1.8	1.8
170	1.7	1.8	1.8	1.8	1.8	1.8	1.9
180	1.8	1.8	1.8	1.9	1.9	1.9	1.9
190	1.8	1.9	1.9	1.9	1.9	1.9	2.0
200	1.9	1.9	1.9	1.9	2.0	2.0	2.0
210	1.9	1.9	2.0	2.0	2.0	2.0	2.0
220	1.9	2.0	2.0	2.0	2.0	2.1	2.1
230	2.0	2.0	2.0	2.1	2.1	2.1	2.1
240	2.0	2.0	2.1	2.1	2.1	2.1	2.2
250	2.1	2.1	2.1	2.1	2.2	2.2	2.2
260	2.1	2.1	2.1	2.2	2.2	2.2	2.2
270	2.1	2.1	2.2	2.2	2.2	2.2	2.3
280	2.2	2.2	2.2	2.2	2.3	2.3	2.3
290	2.2	2.2	2.2	2.3	2.3	2.3	2.3
300	2.2	2.2	2.3	2.3	2.3	2.4	2.4
310	2.3	2.3	2.3	2.3	2.4	2.4	2.4
320	2.3	2.3	2.3	2.4	2.4	2.4	2.4
330	2.3	2.3	2.4	2.4	2.4	2.4	2.5
340	2.3	2.4	2.4	2.4	2.5	2.5	2.5
350	2.4	2.4	2.4	2.5	2.5	2.5	2.5

Source: Generated by Ross Andersen, Ph.D., based on the Robertson and Reid (1952) equation recently validated as an accurate predication equation for resting energy expenditure in an obese sample. Stanley Heshka, Kathy Feld, and Mei-Uih Yang, "Resting Energy Expenditure in the Obese: A Cross-Validation and Comparison of Predication Equations," *Journal of the American Dietetic Association* 93, no. 9 (September 1993): 1031–36.

			Height (Inches)				
67	68	69	70	71	72	73	74
1.5	1.5	1.5	1.6	1.6	1.6	1.6	1.6
1.6	1.6	1.6	1.6	1.6	1.7	1.7	1.7
1.6	1.6	1.7	1.7	1.7	1.7	1.7	1.8
1.7	1.7	1.7	1.7	1.8	1.8	1.8	1.8
1.7	1.8	1.8	1.8	1.8	1.8	1.9	1.9
1.8	1.8	1.8	1.8	1.9	1.9	1.9	1.9
1.8	1.9	1.9	1.9	1.9	1.9	2.0	2.0
1.9	1.9	1.9	1.9	2.0	2.0	2.0	2.0
1.9	2.0	2.0	2.0	2.0	2.0	2.1	2.1
2.0	2.0	2.0	2.0	2.1	2.1	2.1	2.1
2.0	2.0	2.1	2.1	2.1	2.1	2.2	2.2
2.1	2.1	2.1	2.1	2.2	2.2	2.2	2.2
2.1	2.1	2.2	2.2	2.2	2.2	2.2	2.3
2.1	2.2	2.2	2.2	2.2	2.3	2.3	2.3
2.2	2.2	2.2	2.3	2.3	2.3	2.3	2.4
2.2	2.2	2.3	2.3	2.3	2.3	2.4	2.4
2.3	2.3	2.3	2.3	2.4	2.4	2.4	2.4
2.3	2.3	2.3	2.4	2.4	2.4	2.4	2.5
2.3	2.4	2.4	2.4	2.4	2.5	2.5	2.5
2.4	2.4	2.4	2.4	2.5	2.5	2.5	2.5
2.4	2.4	2.5	2.5	2.5	2.5	2.6	2.6
2.4	2.5	2.5	2.5	2.5	2.6	2.6	2.6
2.5	2.5	2.5	2.6	2.6	2.6	2.6	2.7
2.5	2.5	2.6	2.6	2.6	2.6	2.7	2.7
2.5	2.6	2.6	2.6	2.6	2.7	2.7	2.7
2.6	2.6	2.6	2.7	2.7	2.7	2.7	2.8

TABLE 6.3 FEMALE RMR PREDICTIONS (KCAL/D)
BSA Taken from Table 6.2

Age	1.4	1.5	1.6	1.7	1.8	1.9
15	1236	1325	1413	1501	1590	1678
16	1210	1296	1382	1469	1555	1642
17	1186	1271	1356	1440	1525	1610
18	1173	1256	1340	1424	1508	1591
19	1159	1242	1325	1408	1490	1573
20	1152	1235	1317	1399	1482	1564
22	1142	1224	1306	1387	1469	1550
24	1139	1220	1302	1383	1464	1546
26	1142	1224	1306	1387	1469	1550
28	1142	1224	1306	1387	1469	1550
30	1146	1228	1309	1391	1473	1555
32	1139	1220	1302	1383	1464	1546
34	1132	1213	1294	1375	1456	1537
36	1119	1199	1279	1359	1439	1518
38	1105	1184	1263	1342	1421	1500
40	1095	1174	1252	1330	1408	1487
41–44	1092	1170	1248	1326	1404	1482
45–49	1082	1159	1236	1314	1391	1468
50–54	1072	1148	1225	1302	1378	1455
55–59	1062	1138	1213	1289	1365	1441
60–64	1052	1127	1202	1277	1352	1427
65–69	1042	1116	1190	1265	1339	1414
70–74	1032	1105	1179	1253	1326	1400
75 or more	1021	1094	1167	1240	1313	1386

Source: Generated by Ross Andersen, Ph.D., based on the Robertson and Reid (1952) equation recently validated as an accurate predication equation for resting energy expenditure in an obese sample. Stanley Heshka, Kathy Feld, and Mei-Uih Yang, "Resting Energy Expenditure in the Obese: A Cross-Validation and Comparison of Predication Equations," *Journal of the American Dietetic Association* 93, no. 9 (September 1993): 1031–36.

2.0	2.1	2.2	2.3	2.4	2.5	2.6	2.7
1766	1855	1943	2031	2120	2208	2296	2385
1728	1814	1901	1987	2074	2160	2246	2333
1694	1779	1864	1949	2033	2118	2203	2287
1675	1759	1843	1926	2010	2094	2178	2262
1656	1739	1822	1904	1987	2070	2153	2236
1646	1729	1811	1893	1976	2058	2140	2223
1632	1714	1795	1877	1958	2040	2122	2203
1627	1709	1790	1871	1953	2034	2115	2197
1632	1714	1795	1877	1958	2040	2122	2203
1632	1714	1795	1877	1958	2040	2122	2203
1637	1719	1800	1882	1964	2046	2128	2210
1627	1709	1790	1871	1953	2034	2115	2197
1618	1698	1779	1860	1941	2022	2103	2184
1598	1678	1758	1838	1918	1998	2078	2158
1579	1658	1737	1816	1895	1974	2053	2132
1565	1643	1721	1800	1878	1956	2034	2112
1560	1638	1716	1794	1872	1950	2028	2106
1546	1623	1700	1777	1855	1932	2009	2087
1531	1608	1684	1761	1837	1914	1991	2067
1517	1593	1668	1744	1820	1896	1972	2048
1502	1578	1653	1728	1803	1878	1953	2028
1488	1562	1637	1711	1786	1860	1934	2009
1474	1547	1621	1695	1768	1842	1916	1989
1459	1532	1605	1678	1751	1824	1897	1970

TABLE 6.4 MALE RMR PREDICTIONS (KCAL/D)
BSA Taken from Table 6.2

Age	1.4	1.5	1.6	1.7	1.8	1.9
15	1378	1476	1574	1673	1771	1870
16	1354	1451	1548	1644	1741	1838
17	1334	1429	1524	1620	1715	1810
18	1317	1411	1505	1599	1693	1788
19	1304	1397	1490	1583	1676	1769
20	1290	1382	1475	1567	1659	1751
22	1270	1361	1452	1542	1633	1724
24	1253	1343	1432	1522	1611	1701
26	1243	1332	1421	1510	1598	1687
28	1230	1318	1405	1493	1581	1669
30	1223	1310	1398	1485	1572	1660
32	1216	1303	1390	1477	1564	1651
34	1210	1296	1382	1469	1555	1642
36	1203	1289	1375	1461	1547	1632
38	1200	1285	1371	1457	1542	1628
40	1193	1278	1363	1448	1534	1619
41–44	1159	1242	1325	1408	1490	1573
45–49	1146	1228	1309	1391	1473	1555
50–54	1136	1217	1298	1379	1460	1541
55–59	1122	1202	1283	1363	1443	1523
60–64	1112	1192	1271	1350	1430	1509
65–69	1099	1177	1256	1334	1413	1491
70–74	1089	1166	1244	1322	1400	1477
75 or more	1075	1152	1229	1306	1382	1459

Source: Generated by Ross Andersen, Ph.D., based on the Robertson and Reid (1952) equation recently validated as an accurate predication equation for resting energy expenditure in an obese sample. Stanley Heshka, Kathy Feld, and Mei-Uih Yang, "Resting Energy Expenditure in the Obese: A Cross-Validation and Comparison of Predication Equations," *Journal of the American Dietetic Association* 93, no. 9 (September 1993): 1031–36.

2.0	2.1	2.2	2.3	2.4	2.5	2.6	2.7
1968	2066	2165	2263	2362	2460	2558	2657
1934	2031	2128	2225	2321	2418	2515	2611
1906	2001	2096	2191	2287	2382	2477	2573
1882	1976	2070	2164	2258	2352	2446	2540
1862	1956	2049	2142	2235	2328	2421	2514
1843	1935	2028	2120	2212	2304	2396	2488
1814	1905	1996	2087	2177	2268	2359	2449
1790	1880	1969	2059	2148	2238	2328	2417
1776	1865	1954	2042	2131	2220	2309	2398
1757	1845	1932	2020	2108	2196	2284	2372
1747	1835	1922	2009	2097	2184	2271	2359
1738	1824	1911	1998	2085	2172	2259	2346
1728	1814	1901	1987	2074	2160	2246	2333
1718	1804	1890	1976	2062	2148	2234	2320
1714	1799	1885	1971	2056	2142	2228	2313
1704	1789	1874	1960	2045	2130	2215	2300
1656	1739	1822	1904	1987	2070	2153	2236
1637	1719	1800	1882	1964	2046	2128	2210
1622	1704	1785	1866	1947	2028	2109	2190
1603	1683	1764	1844	1924	2004	2084	2164
1589	1668	1748	1827	1907	1986	2065	2145
1570	1648	1727	1805	1884	1962	2040	2119
1555	1633	1711	1788	1866	1944	2022	2100
1536	1613	1690	1766	1843	1920	1997	2074

TABLE 6.5 TOTAL DAILY ENERGY NEEDS

RMR (kcal/d)	Activity Factor		
	1.3	1.5	1.7
1000	1300	1500	1700
1050	1365	1575	1785
1100	1430	1650	1870
1150	1495	1725	1955
1200	1560	1800	2040
1250	1625	1875	2125
1300	1690	1950	2210
1350	1755	2025	2295
1400	1820	2100	2380
1450	1885	2175	2465
1500	1950	2250	2550
1550	2015	2325	2635
1600	2080	2400	2720
1650	2145	2475	2805
1700	2210	2550	2890
1750	2275	2625	2975
1800	2340	2700	3060
1850	2405	2775	3145
1900	2470	2850	3230
1950	2535	2925	3315
2000	2600	3000	3400
2050	2665	3075	3485
2100	2730	3150	3570
2150	2795	3225	3655
2200	2860	3300	3740
2250	2925	3375	3825
2300	2990	3450	3910

Source: Generated by Ross Andersen, Ph.D., based on the Robertson and Reid (1952) equation recently validated as an accurate predication equation for resting energy expenditure in an obese sample. Stanley Heshka, Kathy Feld, and Mei-Uih Yang, "Resting Energy Expenditure in the Obese: A Cross-Validation and Comparison of Predication Equations," *Journal of the American Dietetic Association* 93, no. 9 (September 1993): 1031–36.

TABLE 6.6 PYRAMID PATTERNS FOR HEALTHFUL WEIGHT LOSS AND MAINTENANCE

Food Group	Servings per Total Daily Calories				
	1200–1400	1400–1600	1600–1800	1800–2000	2000–2200
Bread	6	7	8	9	10
Vegetable	3	4	4	5	5
Fruit	2	2	3	3	4
Milk	2	2	2	2	2
Meat	2	2	2	2	2
Fats, Oils, Sweets	0–1	0–2	1–2	1–3	2–3

TABLE 6.7 FAT GRAM TABLE

Calorie Level	Total Daily Fat Grams
1200–1400	20–33
1400–1600	23–39
1600–1800	27–44
1800–2000	30–50
2000–2200	33–56

The Three-Day Dietary Evaluation

Now that you've decided on your daily calories, food selection pattern, and fat budget for losing a certain amount of weight over a given period of time, it's time to evaluate the way you are *currently* eating, to get a sense of what and how much daily change you will need to make to achieve your goals.

For the next three days, eat the same way you normally do, but *write down everything* you eat, all day long, in a Daily Food Record. (See the blank Daily Food Record on page 144; you'll need to make several photocopies before you begin this exercise. Following the blank record is an example of a completed food record.) The following instructions will be your guide in recording and evaluating food intake.

Step 1.
Use one food record per day.

Step 2.
Every time you eat or drink something, write it down immediately. Carrying your food record with you will help ensure that everything is recorded promptly.

Step 3.
Record the time of each eating event in the left-hand column.

Step 4.
Record each food or drink consumed in the middle of the page.

   A. Use one line per food item.
   B. Include information about the amount eaten, the type of food, and the preparation technique.

Step 5.
At the end of three days, using food labels and/or the Pyramid Food Tables for Weight Management beginning on page 217, record the amount of fat and calories for each of the items you consumed. To improve the accuracy of your figures, be sure to compare the amount *you ate* to the *amount listed as a serving* on the food label or in the tables. For example, a food label may indicate that each half-cup serving has 100 calories and 4 fat grams. If you ate 1 cup of the item, then you should record 200 calories and 8 fat grams. If you are unfamiliar with the new nutrition food labels, see "Why Read the Label?" (page 146) for information on how to use them to find serving sizes and fat and calorie content.

There's no question that completing this part of the assessment requires some discipline, but the effort will yield very important information about your eating patterns—it may even reveal information about your food habits that surprises you. Completing the dietary evaluation is crucial for designing your Personal Plan; it will also give you practice in the important weight loss and maintenance skill of *self-monitoring*.

Step 6.
After you have recorded the fat and calorie content of all the foods you ate for all three days, it's time to total each fat and calorie column. On a copy of the Three-Day Daily Intake Grid (pages 148–49), record your three daily fat totals. Add the three *fat* totals together and divide by 3. Do the same for *calories*. This is a good estimate of the *average* number of fat grams and calories that you eat per day. Com-

pare the average calories you ate over these three days with the calorie estimate you calculated for your daily energy needs in Step 2 of the Worksheet for Establishing Goals and Dietary Budgets. Are the numbers close? If not, ask yourself if you were totally accurate in recording what you ate. Did you eat in your usual fashion? Did you record everything? If you did, then you may wish to recalculate Steps 5 to 8 on the worksheet based on this new, *actual* information.

Now, compare and contrast the difference between your usual fat and calorie consumption and the fat and calorie budgets for weight loss that you calculated in your Worksheet.

A. I usually eat an average of _____ calories per day. I need to eat _____ calories per day for weight loss. This is a difference of _____ calories.

B. I usually eat an average of _____ fat grams per day. I need to eat no more than _____ fat grams per day for weight loss. This is a difference of _____ grams of fat.

Step 7.
Look at each of your three food records and, line by line, decide which pyramid group the food belongs in and how many servings of the food you ate. Make three copies of the Pyramid Monitoring Guide (page 150), and shade in the appropriate number of boxes for each day. Shade in one box for each food serving that you ate. Be sure that you shade a box for each food serving in the appropriate category. For example, if you ate 1 cup of cooked green beans, then you should shade 2 boxes in the vegetable group, since half a cup of a cooked vegetable counts as one serving. The following general rules will help you determine what counts as *a single serving*.

General Guidelines for Pyramid Servings

Bread, Cereal, Rice, and Pasta Group
    1 slice regular bread
    1 small dinner roll, biscuit, or muffin
    ½ bagel, sandwich roll, or english muffin
    ½ cup rice, macaroni, or pasta
    1 ounce ready-to-eat cereal
    ½ cup cooked cereal
Vegetable Group
    1 cup raw or leafy vegetables
    ½ cup cooked vegetables

(*Continued on page 147*)

DAILY FOOD RECORD FOR 3-DAY DIETARY EVALUATION

Date _____ Day of week _____

Time	List *All* Food or Drinks and Amounts	Fat in Grams	Calories
		TOTALS	

DAILY FOOD RECORD (EXAMPLE)

Date __3/15/97__   Day of week __Saturday__

Time	List *All* Food or Drinks and Amounts	Fat Grams	Calories
8:00 A.M.	Oatmeal, 1 cup	0	150
	Milk, 2%, ½ cup	3	60
	Banana, 1 large	2	155
	Juice, orange, ½ cup	0	52
10:00 A.M.	Doughnut, yeast, glazed, 1 whole	16	270
	Coffee, black	0	0
12:30 P.M.	Bread, white, 2 slices	2	140
	Peanut butter, 2 Tbsp.	16	186
	Jelly, grape, 2 Tbsp.	0	100
	Chips, potato, 2 oz.	20	300
	Soda, cola, 12 oz.	0	160
	Brownie, with nuts, 1 small	6	97
3:00 P.M.	Pretzels, 2 oz.	2	222
5:30 P.M.	Cheese, american, 2 slices (2 oz.)	18	212
	Crackers, saltines, 3	1	40
	Soda, cola, regular, 12 oz.	0	160
7:00 P.M.	Pork chop, fried, 3 oz.	28	334
	Potato, mashed, homemade, 1 cup	8	222
	Peas, green, cooked, ½ cup	0	67
	Margarine, 1 tsp.	4	34
	TOTALS	126	2961

WHY READ THE LABEL?

To help choose foods that make up a healthful diet. Use the information on the labels to make more informed food choices when you buy food. Keep in mind that no one food can make you healthy—you need a variety every day. The new food labels offer a full course of information. For starters, and for purposes of weight management, focus on the following 3 key pieces of information:

Serving Size

Similar food products now have similar serving sizes, making it easier to compare foods. How does the amount *you eat* compare to the serving size on the label? If you eat less or more than what's listed, you'll have to adjust accordingly. Be aware that the serving size listed on the label is not always the same as a pyramid serving size. Serving sizes are based on the average amounts people actually eat.

Calories

The calories listed on the label are *per serving*. Be aware of how many servings there are per container. Look at the calories to see how a serving of food adds to your daily total.

Nutrition Facts

Serving Size 1/2 cup (114 g)
Servings Per Container 4

Amount Per Serving

Calories 90   Calories from Fat 30

	% Daily Value*
Total Fat 3g	5%
Saturated Fat 0g	0%
Cholesterol 0mg	0%
Sodium 300mg	13%
Total Carbohydrate 13g	4%
Dietary Fiber 3g	12%
Sugars 3g	
Protein 3g	

Vitamin A 80%	•	Vitamin C 60%
Calcium 4%	•	Iron 10%

*Percent Daily Values are based on a 2,000 calorie diet. Your daily values may be higher or lower depending on your calorie needs.

		Calories: 2,000	2,500
Total Fat	Less than	65g	80g
Sat Fat	Less than	20g	25g
Cholesterol	Less than	300mg	300mg
Sodium	Less than	2,400mg	2,400mg
Total Carbohydrate		300g	375g
Fiber		25g	30g

Calories per gram:
Fat 9 • Carbohydrate 4 • Protein 4
Other nutrients may be on some labels

Total Fat

"Total Fat" (in grams) and "Calories from Fat" are both listed on the label. How many fat grams should be eaten each day varies by individual. Know your fat budget (how many grams of fat you should eat per day) and use this information to help balance your food choices. Remember, there are 9 calories per gram of fat. *Calories from fat* helps you see how fatty a food is. Fat plays an important role in a healthful diet, but try to limit it to 15–25% of total calories (15–25 calories out of every 100).

1 small white or sweet potato, or yam

¾ cup vegetable juice

Fruit Group

½ cup chopped, canned, or fresh fruit

1 small to medium piece of whole fruit

¾ cup fruit juice

Milk, Yogurt, and Cheese Group

1 cup fluid milk

8 ounces yogurt

1½ ounces natural cheese

2 ounces processed cheese

Meat, Poultry, Fish, Dry Beans, Eggs, and Nuts Group

2–3 ounces cooked lean meat, poultry, or fish

2 eggs or ½ cup egg substitute

1 cup cooked beans (legumes)

4 tablespoons peanut butter

Fats, Oils, and Sweets

1 tablespoon oil, margarine, butter, or mayonnaise

3 slices of bacon

1 ounce snack chips*

½ slice of cake*

2 cookies*

¼–½ cup ice cream*

1 ounce chocolate candy

The serving sizes and foods included in the fats, oils, and sweets group have been altered from the version distributed by the U.S. Department of Agriculture/Department of Health and Human Services to include many items traditionally considered to be snack- or dessert-type foods. Routinely eating these foods will not be appropriate for a high-nutrient food plan with calories and fat controlled for weight management. Items transferred from the five major food groups are marked with an asterisk (*).

For more detailed information about pyramid servings, refer to the Pyramid Food Tables for Weight Management and the Pyramid Pattern Menus at the end of this book. Each set of the tables corresponds to one of the five major pyramid groups. A sixth table, of fats, oils, and sweets, with snack foods and desserts, is also included. The serving size listed for each food item, unless otherwise indicated, is one pyramid serving. Tables for fast foods, ethnic foods, and combination

3-DAY DAILY INTAKE GRID
(for current dietary evaluation)

Day	Number of Servings/Category		
	Bread	Vegetable	Fruit
1			
2			
3			
Total			
Average (Total÷3)			
I Should Eat*			
This is a difference of:			

* Insert budgets for calories, fat, and pyramid pattern.

Number of Servings/Category			Number of Fat Grams	Number of Calories
Milk	Meat	Fats, Oils, Sweets		

PYRAMID MONITORING GUIDE (PMG)
(For 3-Day Dietary Evaluation)
Mark off (shade in, check) a whole box in the appropriate category for each complete serving of food you ate. If you ate only one half of a serving, then shade in only half of a box. If you ate more than is represented by the number of provided boxes, then add additional boxes.

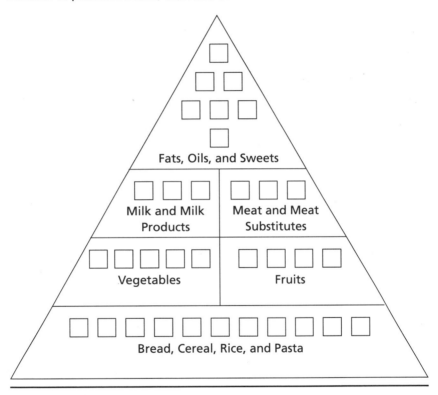

foods are also included. In all tables, **boldface** items *other than* for the five major pyramid groups reflect combination foods whose fat content is less than 30 percent and that can potentially be part of a heart-healthy eating plan for weight control.

Step 8.

After you have completed three Pyramid Monitoring Guides (one for each day), total the number of servings you ate in each of the food groups. Transfer these totals as well as your weight loss budgets (from your Worksheet) to the Three-Day Daily Intake Grid on pages 148–49. Compare these averages with the figures in your budgets for pyramid patterns, fat, and calories.

Step 9.

Review your three daily food records and your Three-Day Daily Intake Grid to decide what changes you would like to make (in hindsight) to bring your eating habits in line with your calculated dietary budgets. Use the following questions to help you make this assessment.

A. Look at the column on the left side of your food records. How often did you eat each day? Did you eat fewer than three times? More than four times? If your answer was fewer than three, and this is a pattern for you, then you may be eating too many calories at a sitting. This pattern of infrequent but high-volume consumption is often associated with difficulty in controlling weight. The related habit of skipping breakfast is harmful because excess hunger or a sense of deprivation can cause you to lose control once you do start eating after a prolonged period of restraint.

If your answer was more than four times, then perhaps you are eating too much by grazing throughout the day. This is a habit many people learn as a way of coping with negative feelings such as stress, fatigue, boredom, loneliness, or pain. Grazing is usually a means of experiencing temporary pleasure and is rarely associated with true physical hunger. Eating food when you are not truly hungry is the perfect activity for *gaining* weight. See Chapter 5 for hints to help you change these inappropriate eating patterns.

B. Look at each eating event. Try to recall the experience. Do you remember feeling hungry? The kind of hunger that's in your stomach, or makes you tremble, or causes lightheadedness or a headache? If each day you felt true physical hunger only once, or not at all, then the chances are very good that your reasons for eating are rarely associated with physical need, and that you eat out of habit or desire. It will be important for you to be reintroduced to the sensation of physical hunger, learn to respond to it in a measured fashion, and plan ahead for its return. You can do this by arranging to eat a meal (light or moderate) within two hours of waking each day and then planning on two or three light to moderate meals or snacks every three to four hours thereafter.

It's usually best not to eat during the two hours before you go to bed. This will allow your appetite to return promptly in the morning and can help you stay on track. Of course if you've missed a meal along the way and you're truly hungry right before bed, then by all means eat something; but try to keep it light—just enough to take the edge off.

C. Now look again at each food record and its companion Pyramid Monitoring Guide. Where are your extra calories coming from?

1. Are there two or more boxes checked off in the tip of the pyramid? If so, then put a line through these items on your daily food record. At the same time, deduct their fat and calories from your daily totals. Note how much difference this makes. Look carefully at these eliminated foods. Ask yourself if you can live without them for awhile, or whether you can eat a much smaller amount of them or eat them less frequently. Alternatively, is there something you can substitute that may be lower in calories and fat that you can eat in the same amount?

2. Moving down each Pyramid Monitoring Guide, what do you see in the milk and meat groups? Are you eating more servings than you budgeted for weight loss? If the answer is yes, then again draw a line through each of the extra portions you ate in these two categories and deduct their fat and calories from the totals in the daily records. Notice how much closer you're getting to your calorie and fat budgets? Apart from portions, another point to consider in these two categories is what foods you're eating. Many high-protein, high-calcium foods (meats and milk) are also very high in fat!

Consider each of the foods you chose to eat in these two categories. Can you think of nutritious alternatives you could have chosen which you might like just as well but which don't pack the same calorie or fat punch? Review the Pyramid Food Tables at the end of the book. Note that some foods are in **boldface type.** These food choices are the lowest in fat. You will also find items that are both in **boldface** and in *italic.* These items are low in both fat *and* calories (or are calorically exchangeable). You may be impressed by the number of delicious foods you can eat while keeping fat and calories within reasonable limits. These tend also to be the most nutrient-dense foods. You can use these tables and the boldface options to help you make the best choices when deciding what to eat, during both weight loss and maintenance. Replace any high-fat meats or high-fat milk products which you're currently eating with lower fat and lower calorie options from the tables. Adjust your daily totals accordingly.

3. Moving further down each Pyramid Monitoring Guide, look at the vegetable and fruit groups. If you're like most people, you didn't eat enough of these foods; you should be eating a minimum of 2 fruits and 3 vegetables, in accord with the National Cancer Institute's "five-a-day for better health" campaign. On each of your three daily records, add enough vegetables and/or fruit servings to bring your servings up to your pyramid pattern goal. Add their respective calories and fat to the totals each day. Note how little fat, if any, you had to add back; calories have gone back up a little, perhaps, but these are calories from carbohydrate, which, you'll recall, are difficult to store as body fat. Chances are good that, so far, you've eliminated some servings of food from the first three groups you looked at, but you've replaced some or all of these foods with servings from bulky, filling fruits and vegetables. Note that little if any food *volume* has been sacrificed, only fat and calories.

4. Now look at the base of the pyramid on your Pyramid Monitoring Guides. Again, if you're like many people, you may not have eaten enough breads, cereals, rice, or pasta. In other words, your Pyramid Monitoring Guides—and your usual diet—may be topheavy. Just as in the fruit and vegetable categories, most but not all foods in this group are very low in fat. It's usually the toppings that turn these into troublesome foods. Adjust each of your food records either up or down to reflect the number of servings you should be eating from this category according to your personal pyramid pattern. If you did eat too many servings, then eliminate just enough to reach your pyramid pattern budget. If your servings are too low, use the food tables to help you add satisfying, low-fat options to your food choices. If you did eat the correct number of servings and some of your choices were high in fat, then replace them with some of the boldface, italic choices (that you like) from the food tables. Adjust your daily totals for fat and calories for each food record accordingly.

D. Now take your three *revised* food records and average the three days together. First add together all three daily calorie totals, then divide by 3. Are the average daily calories close to your calorie goal for weight loss? Now add all three daily fat grams and divide by 3. Are the average fat grams close to your fat gram goals for weight loss? If your answer is No, then review Steps 9A–9D, again using the food tables at the end of the book to help you find lower fat and lower calorie alternatives. If your answer is Yes, and your adjusted records are close to your calorie and fat budgets, then you now have a Personal Plan for how many servings of enjoyable, low-fat foods to choose on a daily basis to reach your weight loss goal. You will be eating satisfying, yet nutritious low-calorie foods.

Developing Your Personal Plan Food Selection Strategy

This section will help you decide on a strategy to use in selecting food wisely and carefully. Your personal strategy should be based on your level of comfort with details and the amount of time you can devote to the task. Your choices are as follows: You can be a "super analyst," a "partial analyst," or a "non-analyst." Any of these strategies can help you succeed in losing weight. Which one is best for you depends on your personal style of dealing with tasks and problems. Which of these three styles most closely matches your preferred approach?

Style 1: The Super Analyst

"I feel most secure and in control of a situation when I know all the facts. I don't like making decisions with incomplete information. I sometimes delay making decisions I know I should make, not because I'm really undecided, but because I don't want to take a chance that I'll make the wrong decision. I am good at detail work. I sometimes notice things other people don't. I tend to be a perfectionist."

Style 2: The Partial Analyst

"I like to understand the 'why' of things I'm doing and some of the facts, but I don't need all of the facts. I am comfortable with some gray areas but not with completely seat-of-the-pants decision-making. I am pretty good at detail work, but I'm not a real perfectionist."

Style 3: The Non-Analyst

"I make decisions mostly based on how I feel—on gut instinct. I'm comfortable if I don't have every bit of information relevant to the decision. In fact, I dislike having to hear all the so-called facts. If there's something I need to do that I don't have a choice about doing, just tell me what it is and don't bore me with the details. I tend to take things as they come, go with the flow, look at the big picture, and not sweat the details."

If you identified most closely with the first description, you will probably do best with the "super analyst" approach—assuming that you're ready and willing to devote the hour or so a day that this strategy requires. Your second choice would be the "partial analyst" strategy; however, even then you may wish to consider starting with the non-analyst, defined-diet approach while you are deciding whether you are comfortable devoting the needed time to a more analytical approach.

If you identified most closely with the second description, you are best suited to the "partial analyst" approach. You may, if you wish, start with a two-week period of the non-analyst, defined-diet approach to get comfortable with the kind of diet you will be following during the active weight loss phase, then switch to the "partial analyst" approach for further weight loss and maintenance.

If you identified most closely with the third description, you will probably do best with the non-analyst, defined-diet approach. Your second choice, and the one that you will need to adopt in the long run for maintenance, is the "partial analyst" strategy.

Read on for a description of the three basic strategies. You may wish to take notes on the strategy you choose to utilize in your Personal Plan of Action.

The Super Analyst

If you're most comfortable with the super analyst approach to weight loss, here are some steps you can follow to lose weight in a way that best suits your personal style. First, plan on eating no more than three or four times each day. Eat your first meal within two hours of waking. Try to eat only when you're hungry, and practice stopping when you are *no longer hungry, or even well before you feel full.* Continue to choose and record your foods every day using the combined Daily Food Record and Pyramid Monitoring Guide, called the Daily Food Record for Dietary Monitoring (pages 156–57), and the Pyramid Food Tables for Weight Management at the end of the book. Record all foods as you eat them.

Instead of waiting until the end of the day to see if you stayed within your calorie, fat, and pyramid pattern budgets, calculate your fat and calories after *each* meal. Also, rate each meal by determining the number and type of pyramid servings using the Pyramid Monitoring Guide. By tracking as you go along, you can make sure that you meet your high-nutrient food group needs without going over your fat and calorie budgets. In other words, you'll know the number of servings, calories, and fat grams that are left in the day *before* you eat your last meal. This will dictate the size and content of this meal.

In this way, on a day-to-day basis, you can maintain very tight control. If you are like most people, you'll probably eat more on some days than on others. It's really what happens *over time* that counts. If you find that indulgences creep in, don't despair. Each week you can fill out a Seven-Day Daily Intake Grid (pages 158–59) to summarize

DAILY FOOD RECORD FOR DIETARY MONITORING

Name _____

Date _____ Day of Week _____

Fat Budget _____ Calorie Budget _____

	Servings	
Food/Beverage Group	I Should Have	I Had
Bread, Cereal, Rice, & Pasta		
Vegetables		
Fruits		
Milk & Milk Products		
Meat & Meat Products		
Fats, Oils, & Sweets	Minimal	
Noncaloric Beverages	8 - 8 oz. cups	

Fats, Oils, and Sweets

Milk and Milk Products

Meat and Meat Substitutes

Vegetables

Fruits

Bread, Cereal, Rice, and Pasta

Time	Food or Drink	Fat Grams	Calories
		TOTAL	
	% CALORIES FROM FAT		

7-DAY DAILY INTAKE GRID
(for weekly summarizing during weight loss)

Day	Number of Servings/Category		
	Bread	Vegetable	Fruit
1			
2			
3			
4			
5			
6			
7			
Total			
Average (Total÷7)			
I Should Eat*			
This is a difference of:			

* Insert budgets for calories, fat, and pyramid pattern.

Number of Servings/Category			Number of	Number of
Milk	Meat	Fats, Oils, Sweets	Fat Grams	Calories

and average your weekly intake. You may find that, on the average, you're meeting your budgets just fine. In other words, if you overeat on one day, you can compensate on another day.

We suggest that you weigh yourself only one day per week, to avoid frustration. Try to weigh in on the same day each week, at approximately the same time. Weigh yourself without clothing. Record your weekly weight using the Weekly Weigh-In Log (below). If after two weeks you are not meeting your weight loss goal, you will need to do one or more of these three things:

1. Readjust your expectations, particularly if you feel that you are doing all that you can or wish to do.
2. Adjust your personal diet plan. Choose a lower calorie level with a corresponding fat budget and pyramid pattern, but only if you won't feel desperately deprived. Don't dip below 1200 calories if you are a woman or 1500 calories if you are a man.
3. Increase your physical activity. This will burn more calories and create a bigger caloric deficit. You may do this either without further dietary modifications or in conjunction with additional dietary changes.

The Partial Analyst, or "One Step at a Time, Please"

In the role of partial analyst for weight loss you will be making gradual changes in the degree of control and monitoring you use to achieve effective weight management. The first and simplest step is to limit your food choices, using the distribution of servings from the food groups in your personal diet pyramid. If this isn't enough to control your diet, you will take a second step and start monitoring fat intake. If this is still not enough, you will take a third step and begin monitoring both fat and calorie intake. At that point, you will have effectively become a super analyst. These decision steps are described below.

Decision 1: I will eat according to my pyramid pattern. Begin your Personal Plan of Action by deciding to eat according to your personal pyramid pattern, as devised in the Worksheet for Establishing Goals and Dietary Budgets. Plan on eating no more than three or four times per day. Try to eat your first meal within two hours of waking. Practice eating only when you're hungry and stop when you are *no longer hungry, not when you're full.* Each day, use one Daily Food Record for Dietary Monitoring and the Pyramid Food Tables for Weight

WEEKLY WEIGH-IN LOG

Name _____

Initial Weight _____   Your Desired Goal Weight _____

Date	Week	Weight	Amount Lost or Gained
	1		
	2		
	3		
	4		
	5		
	6		
	7		
	8		
	9		
	10		
	11		
	12		
	13		
	14		
	15		
	16		
	17		
	18		
	19		
	20		

Reasonable Healthy Weight Range

Dietary Budgets:

Calories _____

Fat Grams _____

Daily Pyramid Pattern:

_____ Bread   _____ Vegetable   _____ Fruit

_____ Milk   _____ Meat   _____ Fats, Oils, Sweets

Management at the end of the book. Record your foods as you eat them in the same way that you did for your three-day evaluation. But, each time you record food eaten, look up how *many* servings you ate in the food tables. Assign your foods to the appropriate category on the PMG part of the form. At this time you *do not* have to record fat and calories. When it's time to eat your last meal of the day, refer to your PMG and determine how many servings from each category you have left. Plan your last meal based on what and how much is left from each category. Use the food tables to help you choose the appropriate types and amount of food to be eaten for this meal.

Repeat this process each day for one or two weeks. At the end of each week, weigh yourself without clothing. Choose the same day each week, weighing in at the same time of day. Record your weight on the Weekly Weigh-In Log. If, after one or two weeks, you are meeting your weight loss goals, then continue monitoring your intake according to your pyramid pattern only. If after two weeks you are not meeting your weight loss goal, proceed to the next decision step.

Decision 2: I will limit total fat. In addition to adhering to your personal pyramid pattern, begin tracking fat grams based on your personal fat budget (Steps 7 and 8, worksheet). Each day for the next one or two weeks (weeks 3 and 4), continue recording and rating all food intake on the food record and corresponding PMG. Additionally, you can use the Pyramid Food Tables at the end of the book to track fat grams. Total your fat grams daily. Transfer the number of pyramid servings and fat grams you ate daily to the Weekly Intake Grid. At the end of one week, you will be able to average your results and compare them with your goals. Record your weight.

On average, did you find that you met your goals? If not, and you didn't lose weight, then try to make an extra effort to adhere to either your pyramid or your fat budget, or both, for the fourth week. If you met your budgets and have lost enough weight to meet your weight loss goal, then continue this strategy of fat budgeting within the context of your pyramid pattern. If you are unsuccessful at weight loss despite your best efforts and compliance, then proceed to the third decision step.

Decision 3: I will reduce total calories. Add calorie counting (steps 5 and 8, worksheet) to fat budgeting and following your pyramid pattern. Refer back to Style 1, "The Super Analyst," for instructions, since you are now in that category.

The Non-Analyst, or "Show Me the Way"

On pages 243–59 you'll find five Pyramid Pattern Menus, which are pre-organized daily menus. Each menu corresponds to a particular calorie range: 1200–1400, 1400–1600, 1600–1800, and 2000–2200. For simplicity and convenience, you can choose and follow a menu based on your personal calorie budget (steps 5 and 8, worksheet). The daily pattern of food options corresponds to the correct pyramid pattern and fat budget for that calorie range (steps 6, 7, and 8, worksheet). Most foods within a pyramid menu food category are roughly equivalent to one another in fat and calories and were chosen based on familiarity, bulk, preference, and convenience. The idea on any given day is to glance down the appropriate meal or snack column and choose the recommended number of servings from each food group in that column. Be careful to follow the portion size as precisely as possible and follow the "key points" at the bottom of the page to ensure a *weekly average* of caloric intake necessary to achieve your weight loss goals. Each food category has five to seven options, so if you vary your choices each day, you will have a satisfying array of daily combinations. Be creative by combining and preparing your food allowances together with a variety of herbs, spices, and low-fat cooking techniques. The rest of this chapter contains helpful tips for buying and preparing food and for eating out.

If the limited options on your daily menu become tedious, turn to the Pyramid Food Tables for Weight Management. Note that within each of the five major groups some of the foods are in boldface type. These designate the low-fat options within the group. The foods that are both in boldface *and* in italic are exchangeable items (in terms of both fat and calories) for the items in boldface on your preplanned menu.

Weigh yourself only one day per week; stay with the same day each week, weighing in at approximately the same time, without clothing. Record your weight on the Weekly Weigh-in Log. If after one to two weeks you are not losing the desired amount of weight despite your best efforts, then you can either step down to the next lower calorie level and its associated menu or increase physical activity, or both. You may also want to review the Worksheet for Establishing Goals and Dietary Budgets on pages 129–33 for possible errors.

Staying the Course in the Real World

Presumably, if you've worked your way through the book to this point, you're well on your way to developing a new way of eating for weight loss based on sound, healthful eating habits. After you've completed your active weight loss phase (within 5 pounds of your ultimate goal weight), gradually increase your total daily calories by 100-200 calories each week until you are no longer losing weight. Choose your foods based on the associated fat budget and pyramid pattern for each new calorie level. This is your maintenance level. Plan to continue eating indefinitely according to your maintenance budgets—at least most of the time.

If you change your habits and lose weight, but then go back to your old way of eating, you will wind up with a frustrating result: weight regain. It's possible that you'll go back up to your former weight, or even higher. Does this mean you can't ever deviate from your plan? Of course not. Just keep in mind that *frequently* deviating from your maintenance plan will result in your gaining weight.

Buying and Preparing Food

If you are one of those people who doesn't take the time to prepare food because you don't like to or because it's time consuming, then you may want to consider the following ideas for storing and preparing food according to pyramid principles with the least amount of effort. Foods marked with an asterisk (*) should be chosen carefully to limit sodium to the recommended maximum of 2400–3000 mg/day, and less if you have hypertension (consult your personal physician).

1. Pasta is a quick and easy meal to fix and can be finished in the time it takes to boil the water and cook the noodles. (No salt or oil in the water, please!) Top with a low-fat bottled marinara sauce*, sprinkle with parmesan cheese, and serve with a pre-mixed, bagged salad tossed with a low-fat salad dressing. If desired, boil a skinless chicken breast simultaneously, chop it up, and add it to the sauce for a pseudo-chicken parmesan.

2. Whip up a batch of vegetarian chili—several boxed mixes* are now available and easy to prepare. Serve with french bread, quick-cooking brown rice, spaghetti, or ears of corn.

3. Make your own pizza. Use pre-made pizza crusts and canned pizza sauce*. Top with pre-shredded low-fat mozzarella and parmesan cheese and any vegetables you desire.

4. Cook up low-fat or fat-free hot dogs* or reduced-fat kielbasa-type sausage* (be careful with the portion size). Serve on buns with sautéed (in cooking spray) onions and green peppers and/or top with leftover vegetarian chili. Serve with microwaved frozen spinach or green peas.

5. Make an omelet—or fake it and scramble all your ingredients in the pan. Use 2 whole eggs, egg substitute, or 2 egg whites with one egg yolk—you decide, based on your fat budget and blood cholesterol level. Fill with your choice of vegetables (peppers, onions, broccoli, spinach, etc.). Sprinkle on some shredded reduced-fat cheese. Serve with toast or a baked potato and enjoy.

6. Buy flour tortillas, canned black beans (rinse before use)*, quick-cooking brown rice, canned chopped green chilis, reduced-fat cheese, low-fat plain yogurt, and salsa*. You'll have the fixings for a good, spicy burrito.

7. Soup's on! You have a few quick choices here. You can open a can of ready-made soup* (preferably clear broth and mostly vegetable) and leave it at that, *or* dilute condensed tomato soup with skim milk adding fresh or frozen spinach for color and nutrients, *or* buy low-sodium chicken broth and add whatever's in your refrigerator—leftover turkey, chicken, vegetables, rice, pasta, etc. Serve with crackers or bread.

8. Stir-fry! In a nonstick skillet coated with cooking spray, quickly brown lightly floured chicken pieces or shrimp. Add soy sauce*, low-sodium chicken broth, ginger, and garlic to taste. Add your choice of vegetables (peppers, onions, broccoli, carrots, cauliflower, etc.) and bring to a boil. Cover and simmer until vegetables are tender-crisp. Serve over quick-cooking brown rice.

9. Pop and top—a potato, that is. Large Idaho potatoes microwave in 4 to 10 minutes. (Pierce them several times with a fork first.) Top with leftover stir-fry or vegetarian chili, reduced-fat cheddar cheese, and low-fat yogurt for a one-dish meal.

10. Brown bag creatively. Make extra of any of the above to take to work. Just package it up the night before while you're cleaning up dinner—then it's just a matter of remembering to grab the container as you leave the house the next day.

Your Personal Plan will be easier to follow if you stock your pantry according to pyramid guidelines. To make sure that you get home from the grocery store with appropriate foods, try a shopping cart analysis. Take your usual trip to the grocery store this week. Buy *food items only*. Organize your shopping list according to the pyramid groups. As you go through the store, treat your grocery cart as if it were the pyramid by placing foods from the bottom portion of the pyramid (breads and grains, vegetables, and fruits) in the main basket (largest part) of the cart. Place foods from the top portion of the pyramid (milk and milk products, meat and meat substitutes, and fats, oils, and sweets) in the child's seat. Place combination foods in the part of the cart which best represents the product.

When you get to the checkout line, take a moment to look at the balance of foods in your cart. If the child's seat is overflowing with items, or has more in it than the main basket, it's time to take a closer look at the Food Guide Pyramid and the nutrition facts panel ("Why Read the Label?") and think about what your choices offer in terms of nutrient balance, volume, proportion, and calorie content. Also, consider the simple sugar and sodium content of your choices. Make changes as needed to have a better balanced, low-fat pyramid cart. A pantry stocked according to the pyramid guidelines helps you to eat within your fat and calorie budgets and your personal pyramid pattern.

Keep in mind that grocery stores are a lot like TV ads: they're designed to encourage you to spend your money impulsively by appealing to your senses and your desire for convenience. The following lists of Dos and Don'ts may help you translate pyramid wisdom into grocery store purchases.

The Top 10 List of Shopping Dos and Don'ts

1. Do make a list. Without a list, you'll waste time, forget necessary items, and indulge in impulse buying. Making a list will force you to get organized. When your cupboard is well stocked with the ingredients for preparing wholesome meals, you're more likely to make and eat them.

2. Don't be shortsighted. Coupons are great, but only for items from the five basic pyramid groups. Avoid using coupons for high-fat or high–simple sugar versions of the five main groups. It's nice to save money, but not at the expense of putting on extra pounds.

3. Do enjoy perimeter shopping, but limit your time there. Though the outer edges of the store (deli, bakery, salad bar) is where you'll find most of the freshest pyramid basics like bread, bagels, fruit, vegetables, milk, cheese, poultry, and fish, these areas also offer many appealing, expensive, high-fat foods. For instance, the deli is great for freshly sliced lean sandwich ham, but it's also the home of six varieties of potato salad or macaroni salad drenched in oil or mayonnaise. So, be careful to stick to your list of appropriate pyramid foods while shopping these hot spots.

4. Don't shop haphazardly. Poor planning results in disorganization, and may even propel you to the fast food window! Follow a routine, choosing a time when you are relaxed and have had a satisfying, healthful meal. You'll be more likely to remain organized and focused, and leave the store with sensible choices.

5. Do compare items on your list by both price and nutritional value. Don't buy low-fat junk foods if they don't fit into your calorie and fat budgets. Remember, fat-free is *not* calorie-free. Be just as careful with newly formulated foods with fat replacers—they can have undesirable side effects. Familiarize yourself with food labels (see page 146) to get the best nutritional bang (with the fewest calories) for your buck.

6. Don't toss purchases into your cart randomly. Organize your purchases. Shop from your list, making conscious decisions based on price, nutrition, and taste. Don't forget to arrange items in your cart according to the pyramid groups. This will give you a clearer picture of your choices for last-minute buying changes.

7. Do spend much of your shopping trip in the produce department. Choose as many richly colored items (dark green, orange, yellow, red) as possible. Most people do not eat the recommended "5-a-day" of fruits and vegetables and cite price or time as barriers. Knowing what's in season and taking a little time to comparison shop will help you pick out excellent nutrition for the best price. For convenience (if price isn't your most pressing consideration), choose prewashed, peeled, chopped, ready-to-eat or pre-assembled options like baby carrots, bagged tossed salads, slaw mixtures, and (of course) cut-up, prepackaged fresh fruit. If you can't find an item on your list, or it doesn't appear fresh, or the price is outrageous, look for a reasonable alternative. (Consider that many people forgo a $1.49 cantaloupe but never blink an eye at a $2.99 bag of potato chips.) Don't be so easily dissuaded from making the more nutritious purchase.

8. Don't skip calcium-rich foods, particularly if you're a woman. With low-fat milk products in abundance, there is no reason to snub these important foods, which help prevent osteoporosis. There are many varieties of low-fat cheese, yogurt, and other milk products, and their taste and texture have been steadily improving. If you are lactose intolerant, choose fermented or lactase-treated milk products. Sometimes small amounts of lactose-rich foods (pyramid portions) are well tolerated even when large amounts are not. For those of you who refuse dairy products for personal reasons, look carefully for calcium-rich substitutes. Many soy products and some cereals and fruit juices are fortified with calcium.

9. Do beware of interior aisles. Don't get trapped by enticing displays for inappropriate foods inside or at the ends of the aisles. If your list doesn't necessitate cruising every aisle, don't! Remember, though, that fruits, vegetables, breads, and grains come in a variety of forms found in interior aisles (canned or frozen vegetables, rice, juice, etc.). These may be just as nutritious as their fresh counterparts—and, sometimes, depending on the time of year, less expensive.

10. Don't be tempted to buy fresh meat, poultry, and fish indiscriminately. These foods are expensive, and many are not yet mandated to have a nutrition facts panel on the package. When information is unavailable, use these rules to help: White meat poultry is leaner than dark; skinless is leaner than skin-on (you can remove the skin yourself); red meats closely trimmed of outer-layer fat are preferred; red meats are leanest if flecks of white between red muscle (known as marbling) are minimal; prime cuts are fattiest, round and loin are leanest; intact cuts of meat or poultry tend to be leaner than ground; and pre-breaded chops, chicken, and fish can often be high in both fat and sodium. Choose white meat poultry, lean pork, and fish much more often than beef. Keep in mind that 4 ounces (¼ lb.) of raw meat will yield 2-3 ounces of cooked, which is a pyramid serving. Even if the meat is lean, try not to eat meats at every lunch and dinner meal. Substituting nuts, seeds, and beans can increase variety and enjoyment while improving the overall nutrition profile of your sensible food plan. Don't worry about getting enough protein. Most Americans eat more than 2 to 3 times the protein they need. Meals based on vegetables and grains can supply you with plenty of protein while increasing fiber and minimizing cholesterol and saturated fat.

Eating Out

While you're actively losing weight, it's best that you prepare your own meals as much as possible. Eating away from home is generally incompatible with weight loss, and can sabotage maintenance. Here's why:

1. You can't monitor the fat and calorie content of restaurant food.
2. In restaurants, portions are almost always larger than you would serve yourself. Restaurant portions have been getting

even larger in recent years. (Even foods like bagels are getting bigger and bigger.) The temptation to eat the whole thing can be overwhelming.

3. Even though people are eating out more than ever before, they still tend to regard the occasion as a reward or celebration, often exercising less than their usual restraint in what they order and consume.

After you have lost weight and are working on maintaining your new weight, it is possible to eat away from home more frequently, as long as control strategies are in place. Dietary control strategies for eating out can be divided into three phases: before, during, and after the event.

Before going out, follow these tips:

- Eat regular meals. Do *not* skip meals prior to eating out, or you may be tempted to "celebrate" your earlier restraint. If you plan to overindulge, eat lightly, but *do* eat something at the usual mealtime prior to the one eaten out.
- Call the restaurant or event planner and ask about the menu. Find out if they accommodate requests for fat-free or low-fat items and methods of preparation. If you are going to someone's home, ask if you can bring a dish (something you know you can eat) or find out if the host or hostess can accommodate your needs.
- Just before going out, have a low-fat snack or a glass of juice to help control unexpected, intense hunger between ordering and receiving the meal.

While you are out, try the following:

- Try not to fill up on the "freebies" put on the table before your food order arrives. You can ask for these items to be eliminated or removed. If you do decide to eat the bread, however, eat it without the butter. *Avoid* tortilla chips—they're fried. If it's a cracker basket, choose saltines or melba toast; the other crackers tend to be higher in fat and calories.
- Resist ordering an appetizer unless it's a low-fat soup or salad, or a shrimp or seafood cocktail. Most other appetizers are fried or loaded with high-fat cheese.
- Minimize alcohol consumption. Alcohol is high in calories, lowers your inhibitions so that you may eat more than you intended, and temporarily shuts down the burning of fat.

- When choosing what to order, avoid fried foods, cream sauces and gravies, large slabs of red meat, sour cream, and butter or margarine.
- Also avoid foods with descriptions like *au gratin, scalloped, cream of.*
- When ordering, ask that the food be broiled rather than fried. In many restaurants, however, liquid fat is poured over food before it is "broiled." To avoid this, ask that it be broiled *without fat.* (Chicken, fish, crab cakes, and other foods can be broiled with water, lemon juice, or broth.)
- Order foods that are lower in fat—fish and chicken, for example, rather than pork or beef (keep preparation in mind); baked or boiled potatoes rather than french fries; tossed salad instead of coleslaw; fresh fruit instead of cheesecake.
- Ask that all dressings, condiments, gravies, and sauces be served *on the side,* so you can control how much you use. If a fat-free, low-calorie salad dressing is unavailable, order the regular on the side, dip your fork in the dressing first, and then spear a bite of salad. This cuts down dramatically on the amount of dressing used. Fresh lemon juice and red wine vinegar are also tasty on a salad. They can be used alone or to stretch a high-fat dressing.
- Order *a la carte* to avoid a full-course meal that may be too much for you.
- Consider ordering an appetizer-size portion of a favorite entrée.
- Eat half of a large order and take the other half home to enjoy at a later time, or split an order of something with a dining partner.
- *Take your time.* Pay attention to both hunger and satiety signals.
- Don't try to match your dining partner(s) bite for bite. They may be able to eat more than you can. You may feel that this is unfair, but *your needs* are what you should be concentrating on.
- To avoid "picking" and overeating, ask the server to take your plate away as soon as you are finished.
- If dessert is a must, order fruit or sorbet. If only something more fattening will do, then *share.*

After the event, particularly if you ate more than you planned, do the following:

- Eat lightly for the next 24 hours if the meal out was higher in calories than normal.
- Consider building in extra physical activity to help compensate for any extra calories eaten.

- Review any unplanned eating you did and identify why it happened. Plan ways to avoid these problems in the future.

If you want to enjoy eating out, without filling out, you must *plan ahead* and compensate for deviations either before or after the event.

CHOOSING HEALTHFUL FOODS OF ALL TYPES, IN ALL PLACES

Italian
- Pasta is low in fat, but cream, butter, and meat sauces are not. Instead of these sauces, order marinara, clam, or marsala sauces. Control the portion, as well, since calories still add up when portions grow in size.
- Try pasta primavera, chicken cacciatore, or shrimp sautéed in white wine over linguini.
- Avoid meat and cheese lasagna, and dishes made with sausage.
- Go easy on the garlic bread. It's really *butter* bread with some garlic. Eat plain Italian bread instead. You can use it to sop up your low-calorie marinara sauce.
- Enjoy your pizza, but avoid meat toppings, olives, and extra cheese. Try vegetable toppings instead (broccoli, green peppers, onions, carrots, and cauliflower), or fruit toppings like pineapple. If there are pools of oil visible on top of the pizza, soak them up with a folded paper napkin.
- Choose thin crust pizza, which has fewer calories than thick crust pizza.

Mexican
- Order chicken fajitas, black beans, vegetable tacos, soft tacos, or corn tortillas.
- Sour cream, chips, nachos, refried beans, guacamole, and all deep-fried foods such as chimichangas are high in fat and calories and should be eaten only in limited quantities. Salsa, on the other hand, can be poured over anything to add lots of flavor and very few calories.

French
- Poached or steamed dishes can be flavored with wine. Oven-baked herbed chicken or poached salmon with capers are excellent choices.
- Think twice about sauces such as white sauce, hollandaise, bearnaise, or butter sauce. Order sauces on the side. Try

dipping your fork into the rich sauce, then put the fork in your mouth so you get just a taste on your tongue, and follow with a forkful of the entrée without sauce. As with salad dressings, this trick cuts down dramatically on the amount of sauce you will consume while preserving a surprising amount of the taste.

Chinese

- You have a lot to choose from because a wide variety of vegetables are used in Chinese foods, and you can order entrées that are composed primarily of vegetables. If you wish to have meat, choose chicken or fish.
- Avoid fried wontons, egg rolls, twice-fried meat entrées like sweet and sour chicken, and any other fried foods.
- Order clear soups like rice broth.
- Avoid fried rice. Choose steamed white rice instead.
- Ask that all dishes be prepared with as little oil as possible.

American

- Select small, lean cuts of beef from the round or the loin.
- Skip gravy and sauces, including "au jus."
- Have plain baked potatoes. Use *no, or very little, sour cream, butter, or bacon*. Lemon juice and fresh ground pepper are delicious on baked potatoes.
- Avoid fried and cheesy appetizers like zucchini sticks, fried mozzarella sticks, and potato skins. Select clear broth soups, garden salads, or shrimp cocktail instead.

Fast Food

- Eat fast food only at mealtimes, not as snacks.
- Order small burgers with lettuce, onion, ketchup, and mustard, or have roast beef or grilled chicken.
- Avoid mayonnaise-based sauces and ask to be served an unbuttered bun.
- Go easy on the french fries, perhaps splitting a small order with someone else. Blot off excess cooking oil by squeezing the fries gently with a paper napkin.
- Most fast food restaurants offer salads. Take advantage of this, but don't forget to use low-fat dressing or regular dressing (on the side); dip fork as described above.
- Order diet soda, juice, or skim milk. Avoid milkshakes and regular soda.

- For breakfast: avoid egg sandwiches with sausage or bacon. Instead of big breakfast platters, have pancakes and juice, or scrambled eggs with an english muffin. Request unbuttered ("dry") breakfast breads.
- Many fast food outlets will provide printed nutrition information on request, so you can make your choices based on total calories and fat grams as well as personal preference.

Salad Bars
- Salad bars can be wonderful, but go easy on cheese, bacon, croutons, avocados, and sunflower seeds.
- Avoid potato, tuna, seafood, pasta, and macaroni salads. Often, more than 50 percent of their calories are from fat (oil or mayonnaise).
- Use low-fat or fat-free dressings. If you do use regular dressing, use just a little and stretch it with vinegar or lemon juice.

Airline Foods
- Pre-order low-fat or diet meals.
- Bring low-fat, low-calorie foods from home.
- Avoid alcoholic beverages; order tomato juice or diet soda instead. Drink lots of water to prevent dehydration and feeling empty.
- Refuse peanuts or other junk food.
- Remember, you don't have to eat it all or eat it *at* all. Skip dessert.
- Try to stay on your regular eating schedule.
- Bring something to do so you don't get bored.

In this chapter you have been given the tools for developing and practicing a "good" diet. To keep tabs on whether you are still on the path of control, periodically refer to the following list of permanent weight management dietary principles.

Dietary Principles for Permanent Weight Loss and Management

1. Eat a variety of foods in moderation and in proportion to one another. In other words, consistently choose according to your personal pyramid pattern for both portion and calorie control.

2. Eat low-fat foods as often as possible. Budget your fat so that it accounts for less than 30% of total calories (preferably 15–25%).

3. Practice semi-vegetarianism by eating a combined total of at least 5 vegetables and fruits, and 6 servings of bread, cereal, rice, and pasta every day.

4. Choose high-fiber options as often as possible for low-calorie bulk and satiety.

5. Eat fewer foods with added sugars. Avoid junk foods, including fat-free alternatives—they still have many calories and can stall your efforts if you eat too much of them.

6. Eat a minimum of three times per day. Breakfast is essential, although you can wait up to two hours after arising to eat breakfast.

7. Avoid both skipping meals and grazing.

8. Eat only when you are physically hungry, and stop eating when you are no longer hungry. Don't wait to stop eating until you are stuffed. Eat slowly to allow satiety to occur.

9. Plan ahead and backwards. Choose foods for each meal or snack in relation to what you've already eaten that day and what you plan to eat later. Each meal or snack does not stand alone, but rather should be viewed as part of a pattern.

10. Compensate with a little extra calorie reduction or increased physical activity either before or after deviations from your Personal Plan.

You have now successfully developed the dietary aspects of your Personal Plan. The next chapter adds an important nonfood ingredient—physical activity. Perhaps you can devise your individualized Personal Plan so you can eat a bit more but burn it off through enjoyable, health-promoting physical activity. Turn to Chapter 7 to find out how.

SEVEN

Exercise That Works for You

You have now completed the behavior and dietary portions of your Personal Plan of Action. Up to this point, we've focused mainly on the *intake* part of your weight-loss program: what foods to eat, and why. But a complete plan for long-term weight loss and maintenance does not stop there. The *energy burning* side of the equation is a significant factor in weight loss (and gain), as well.

You are undoubtedly all too familiar with how and why you lose or gain weight, but restating the obvious often acts to reinforce a good behavior, so here goes—one more time: *The only way your weight can change is if there is an imbalance between the energy you take in and the energy you use.* If energy intake is greater than energy output, you gain weight. If energy intake is less than energy output, you lose weight.

In most weight loss programs, the focus is on the intake side of this equation. But it is just as valid to lose weight by increasing the energy used. Increasing physical activity while holding energy intake (food consumption) stable is an effective way to lose weight—although not a lot of weight. *The most effective way to lose weight is to combine reduced intake with increased physical activity.* This chapter will explain how to increase output—how to make physical activity an integral part of your Personal Plan.

Why Exercise?

Some people like to exercise. Whether it's bicycling, swimming, running, or aerobic dancing, they enjoy activities that keep them moving. But there are also many people who don't like to exercise. Since it's not something they enjoy, they naturally wonder whether they really need to bother with it. They may wonder whether the benefits of exercise are worth the effort. Finally, they may worry that they're too out of shape to exercise. For these people it's important to explore the benefits of exercise and take a look at different ways to make it more enjoyable.

First, although you can lose weight without exercise, there is a catch. Studies have shown that among people who have lost weight, those who incorporate regular exercise into their lives are more likely to keep the weight off than those who do not. In one study, 90 percent of women who were "maintainers" exercised, compared to only 34 percent of the "regainers." Also, 82 percent of women who said they have never had a weight problem were regular exercisers.

What explains why exercise helps to prevent weight regain? There are probably several factors. Physical activity burns calories, so regular exercisers can get away with a somewhat less restrictive diet and still avoid weight gain. Feeling less deprived probably helps maintain good eating habits. Also, people who incorporate regular exercise into their lives are often more likely to embrace other positive lifestyle changes, such as modification of their eating cues.

If you do manage to incorporate regular exercise into your life, you will be among a small minority of American adults—only one person out of five performs at least 30 minutes of light to moderate physical activity per day. This is not an unreasonable amount of time to devote to one's health, fitness, and weight management. I will discuss some ways to find time in your schedule to include regular exercise.

What are the benefits of regular exercise? In addition to enhancing weight loss and preventing regain, exercise helps reduce the risk of cardiovascular disease, including heart attacks, stroke, high blood pressure, and kidney disease; it reduces blood sugars and "bad" LDL cholesterol; and it increases "good" HDL cholesterol. Also, regular exercise helps strengthen bones and prevent osteoporosis and bone fractures in women.

Aside from the health benefits, there are other benefits to being physically fit. Being able to exert yourself with ease instead of becoming easily winded can make you feel more vibrant, alert, and strong. Many people report improvements in mood, reduction of stress, increased energy, and improved sleep with regular exercise.

What if you are unfit right now and believe that you're not capable of doing much exercise? This can be a sign of a specific medical problem which robs you of strength or endurance (such as heart, lung, or neurologic diseases), or a result of joint problems like arthritis or an injury. If you are out of shape, we recommend that you seek the advice of a physician before embarking on an exercise program, especially if you are over the age of 45 or have a history of medical problems. You should also consult a physician if you have worsening shortness of breath, palpitations, chest pain, or weakness. If you are not sure whether a particular symptom is important, it is best to play it safe and seek medical advice. Below is the Physical Activity Readiness Questionnaire, designed by the British Columbia Ministry of Health to help people decide whether they should see a physician before beginning exercise. Please complete this form and follow its advice.

To reach the point where you get the maximum benefit from exercise, you need to make regular physical activity a part of your life. This constitutes a major lifestyle change for many people. Just like dietary changes, changes in exercise behavior will not help you in the long run if you only do exercise in order to lose weight and do not make it a permanent part of your life. Many people who are overweight and have fairly sedentary lifestyles will not find it easy to do much physical activity at first. They must build their endurance and fitness slowly.

Despite what some fitness centers, exercise equipment manufacturers, and magazine ads claim, it is not possible to use exercise as a way of burning fat in one particular part of the body. You can increase muscle mass in specific areas (your abdomen, for example), but the fat burned when you do abdominal exercises comes from the bloodstream and the entire body, not just from the part being exercised.

While exercise alone cannot accomplish miracles, exercise is an excellent way to make weight loss easier and more likely to last. It should be incorporated into your Personal Plan along with dietary and behavioral change.

The Exercise Self-Assessment

Let's now go through an exercise self-assessment, modeled on the approach we take with patients at the Johns Hopkins Weight Management Center.

The first step is a medical assessment (described in detail in Chapter 3). It's important to see a physician for a medical assessment before you begin a vigorous exercise program. Once you've done that, according to the American College of Sports Medicine, it is generally safe for an apparently healthy adult to begin a moderate-intensity walking program, as long as the person does not have heart, lung, or vascular disease. Regardless of how fit you are or how vigorous your

PHYSICAL ACTIVITY READINESS QUESTIONNAIRE (PAR-Q)

PAR-Q is designed to help you help yourself. Many health benefits are associated with regular exercise, and the completion of PAR-Q is a sensible first step to take if you are planning to increase the amount of physical activity in your life.

For most people physical activity should not pose any problem or hazard. PAR-Q has been designed to identify the small number of adults for whom physical activity might be inappropriate or those who should have medical advice concerning the type of activity most suitable for them.

Common sense is your best guide in answering these few questions. Please read them carefully and check Yes or No opposite each question.

Yes No

____ ____ 1. Has your doctor ever said you have heart trouble?

____ ____ 2. Do you frequently have pains in your heart and chest?

____ ____ 3. Do you often feel faint or have spells of severe dizziness?

____ ____ 4. Has a doctor ever said your blood pressure was too high?

____ ____ 5. Has your doctor ever told you that you have a bone or joint problem such as arthritis that has been aggravated by exercise, or might be made worse with exercise?

____ ____ 6. Is there a good physical reason not mentioned here why you should not follow an activity program even if you wanted to?

____ ____ 7. Are you over age 65 and not accustomed to vigorous exercise?

If you answered *Yes* to one or more questions, and if you have not recently done so, consult with your personal physician by telephone or in person *before* increasing your physical activity and/or taking a fitness test. Tell him or her what questions you answered Yes on PAR-Q, or show him your copy of this form. After medical evaluation, seek advice from your physician as to your suitability for:

unrestricted physical activity, probably on a gradually increasing basis;

restricted or supervised activity to meet your specific needs, at least on an initial basis. Check in your community for special programs or services.

If you answered *No* to all questions, and if you answered PAR-Q accurately, you have reasonable assurance of your present suitability for:

A graduated exercise program: A gradual increase in proper exercise promotes good fitness development while minimizing or eliminating discomfort.

An exercise test: Simple tests of fitness or more complex types may be undertaken if you so desire.

Finally, you should postpone activities if you have a temporary minor illness, such as the common cold.

Source: Developed by the British Columbia Ministry of Health, 1978. Conceptualized and critiqued by the Multidisciplinary Advisory Board on Exercise (MABE). Translation, reproduction, and use in its entirety is encouraged.

exercise program, however, you should stop if the exercise causes pain, shortness of breath, or chest, jaw, or arm discomfort.

When you have the go-ahead from your doctor to proceed, you are ready to take a look at your current level of physical fitness to see where you are starting from. Measuring your current level of fitness precisely and scientifically requires special equipment not available to most individuals. So, we will use your typical level of physical activity as a guide to your overall fitness. To do this, make seven copies of the Self-Assessment Log for Current Physical Activity (page 180), and then record for the past week (or better still, the coming week) all periods of exercise or physical activity in excess of "couch potato" level. Thus, you would record any periods of walking lasting at least 3 minutes (walking to your car doesn't count unless you purposely park at the far end of a large lot), any manual labor such as gardening, vacuuming, or other physical work, any recreational activity that causes you to breathe more deeply and rapidly than a slow walk does, and any periods of planned exercise.

Here's a sample completed time slot:

| Time Slot | Tasks/Activities | Physically Active? | |
		Yes	No
3:00–4:00 P.M.	on phone, 35 minutes; deskwork, 15 minutes; walk to vending machine for candy bar, 3 minutes; talk with co-workers (standing), 7 minutes	3 min.	57 min.

SELF-ASSESSMENT LOG FOR CURRENT PHYSICAL ACTIVITY

Date: _____ Day of Week: _____

Time Slot	Tasks/Activities	Physically Active? Yes	No
A.M.:			
12:00–1:00			
1:00–2:00			
2:00–3:00			
3:00–4:00			
4:00–5:00			
5:00–6:00			
6:00–7:00			
7:00–8:00			
8:00–9:00			
9:00–10:00			
10:00–11:00			
11:00 A.M.–12:00 P.M.			
P.M.:			
12:00–1:00			
1:00–2:00			
2:00–3:00			
3:00–4:00			
4:00–5:00			
5:00–6:00			
6:00–7:00			
7:00–8:00			
8:00–9:00			
9:00–10:00			
10:00–11:00			
11:00 P.M.–12:00 A.M.			

Now, add up the total time for the week and divide by 7 to get your average daily exercise duration. If the week you recorded is not typical, you can repeat the assessment or adjust it to better reflect your typical week. Record that number, your average daily exercise, here: _____ minutes.

Now use the key below to determine your present activity level.

Minutes per Day	Activity Level
0–10	couch potato
11–20	borderline
21–40	active
41 or more	very active

This is just a rough measure, of course. If your time is spent in very vigorous aerobic activity like running, you will be more fit than someone who spends the same amount of time walking. One of the things you will be urged to do in devising the exercise portion of your Personal Plan is to slowly increase the intensity of the physical activity you engage in, so that you will become more fit and burn more calories for a given amount of time committed to physical activity.

Now, imagine you were completing the above activity record earlier in your life, and record your best estimate of the number of minutes you spent on average each day exercising at the following ages (when applicable):

Age 15?   _____ minutes
Age 25?   _____ minutes
Age 35?   _____ minutes
Age 45?   _____ minutes
Age 55?   _____ minutes
Age 65?   _____ minutes

If you're like most people, you will note that the amount of time spent exercising declined as you got older. This is valuable information: it demonstrates that difficulties with weight management may be correlated with decreasing amounts of physical activity. The rise in the proportion of people in white-collar jobs compounds this problem. While there are other factors, for most people lack of exercise is widely believed to be one of the most important factors in weight gain.

Another tidbit of information that can be obtained from examining your current and past levels of physical fitness is to recall the kinds of physical activity you used to enjoy at a younger age. Many people shun exercise because they find it boring. This can certainly be true if you think of exercise only in terms of pedaling an exercise bike in the basement.

On the other hand, many people have fond memories of an earlier age when they felt physically fit and enjoyed sports or other activities. If your favorite activity was playing street hockey with friends, then it may not be safe or practical to resurrect this activity exactly. But you could, for example, join a softball team, or play golf.

Now that we've touched on the subject of enjoyable physical activities, it may be helpful to write down some things that you used to enjoy at another time in your life, and any reasonable substitutes that you could enjoy today.

Former Activity	Updated Substitute Activity
1. _____	_____
2. _____	_____
3. _____	_____

If you're having trouble thinking of activities you used to enjoy, perhaps it will help to think back to your summer breaks while in high school (tennis? skateboarding?), on your vacation (hiking? horseback riding? windsurfing?), or at family get-togethers (horseshoes? volleyball?). What did you do then? Now try again filling in the blanks above. We will use this list of activities later on in your Personal Plan, when you have advanced to a high enough level of fitness to begin broadening the scope of your physical activities.

Many people believe that exercise is beneficial only when it is done vigorously, frequently, and uninterruptedly. For years, exercise scientists and physicians have known that 20 to 60 minutes of moderate to high-intensity activity three or more times every week will optimize both physical fitness and general health. However, the results of recent studies show that you don't have to work as hard as you would in a traditional exercise program to benefit from increased physical activity. Even done at much lower levels of intensity, exercise is good for your health. These findings have prompted the American College of Sports Medicine and the Centers for Disease Control to recommend the following: "Every American adult should accumulate 30 minutes or more of moderate intensity physical activity on most, preferably all, days of the week."

How would you rank your current level of physical activity? Place yourself within one of the following three categories:

1. Sedentary
2. Moderately or irregularly active
3. Regularly active

If you are sedentary, I suggest that you attempt to make small changes over time (an approach that is physically and behaviorally sound). By placing emphasis on accumulating moderately intense physical activity throughout the day you will be painlessly spending calories. Try to make lifestyle activity a part of your daily life.

Table 7.1 presents some examples of the time in minutes required to expend 200 calories with various physical activities. Note that heavier people expend the 200 calories faster than lighter people.

Next, you need to learn how vigorously you should exercise to reap the maximum fitness benefits. The usual way to estimate how much energy you are burning up is to take your pulse while exercising. The higher your pulse (and breathing rate), the more vigorous the activity. If you are untrained or sedentary before you begin to add physical activity to your weight loss program, it is safest to aim for only a moderately fast heart rate during exercise. If you are already physically fit, it is safe to aim for a faster heart rate during exercise.

The heart rate you will aim for is based on your age, your fitness level, and your resting heart rate. To determine your resting heart rate and to monitor your pulse during exercise, you need to learn how to locate your pulse. There are two places you can readily feel your pulse: in your neck and at your wrists. The pulse in the neck is usually the easier to find.

First, place the middle three fingers of your right hand gently in the cleft to the left side of your windpipe. Press the tips of your fingers into the neck and move your fingers around slowly until you locate your pulse. (This is the left carotid artery; you have a carotid artery on both sides of your neck.) The pulse feels like a rhythmic swelling and indicates each time your heart beats and pumps blood through your arteries. Once you have located your pulse, count the number of times you feel it in a 10-second period, using a watch with a second-hand. To convert this to the number of heartbeats per minute, multiply the number by six. Thus, if you feel 15 beats in 10 seconds, your pulse is 15×6, or 90 beats per minute.

The other place to feel your pulse is at the wrist. Place the tips of your three middle fingers lengthwise along the thumb side of your

TABLE 7.1 HOW MANY MINUTES DOES IT TAKE TO CONSUME 200 CALORIES?

Activity	Your Weight, in Pounds		
	100	150	200
Bicycling, slower than 10 mph (light effort)	44	29	22
Aerobic dancing, low impact	53	35	26
Carpet sweeping or sweeping floors	106	70	53
Washing dishes, standing	115	77	57
Carrying groceries upstairs	33	22	17
Food shopping, with cart	75	50	38
Chopping wood	44	29	22
Mowing lawn	48	32	24
Gardening (planting)	66	44	33
Shoveling snow	44	29	22
Jogging	38	25	19
Running, 10 minutes/mile	26	18	13
Running, 8 minutes/mile	21	14	11
Horseback riding	66	44	33
Racquetball, competitive	26	18	13
Volleyball, noncompetitive	88	59	44
Walking, strolling	132	88	66
Walking, moderate pace (3 mph)	75	50	38
Walking, brisk (4.5 mph)	59	39	29
Swimming laps, low to moderate effort	33	22	17
Skating (ice), 9 mph or slower	48	32	24
Skiing (cross country), light effort	38	25	19
Skiing (downhill), light effort	53	35	26

wrist, near the edge, alongside the tendons that cross your wrist (either wrist will do). Again, press down gently and shift your fingers if necessary until you feel a definite pulsation. Then count for ten seconds and calculate your pulse by multiplying the number of beats by 6.

Once you have found your resting (seated, relaxed) pulse rate, you have enough information to calculate your target heart rate. Follow the directions in table 7.2. Be aware that the target heart rate you cal-

TABLE 7.2 CALCULATING YOUR TARGET HEART RATE

	Example	You
1. Start at 220 and subtract your age. (This is your estimated maximum heart rate.)	220 – 44 = 176	220 – ___ = ___
2. Subtract your resting pulse rate (seated).	– 72 = 104	– ___ = ___
3. Choose a target zone. If sedentary, use 60%. If already exercising regularly, use 70 or 75%.	× 70% = 73	× ___ % = ___
4. Add your pulse at rest. This is your exercise target heart rate.	+ 72 = 145	+ ___ = ___
5. Divide the minute rate in number 4 (above) by 6. This is your 10-second target heart rate.	÷ 6 = 24	÷ 6 = ___

culated above is a general guide only. Listen to the signals you receive from your body while you are exercising. If, for example, at the 60 percent target zone you consistently feel that you are not getting a reasonable workout, that you hardly need to breathe any deeper than usual and do not sweat, it may be time for you to move up to the next higher target zone (70 percent). If, on the other hand, you experience severe shortness of breath, dizziness, pain, profuse sweating, a pounding in your chest, or nausea, you should stop exercising immediately. If the symptoms do not go away in short order, seek medical attention immediately. If the symptoms go away quickly when you stop exercising, it is probably still a good idea to consult your physician, but at the least you should heed the message that your body is sending, and slow down.

An alternative way to ensure that you are exercising at an appropriate level of intensity is to use the Rating of Perceived Exertion shown in table 7.3. Working at a level of 12 or 13 is best. At this level of perceived exertion, you should still be able to carry on a conversation while exercising. Using this scale is less precise than measuring your pulse, but it certainly is the easiest way to monitor your exertion level. In fact, however, the most important aspects of exercise for

TABLE 7.3 RATINGS OF PERCEIVED EXERTION

6	
7	Very, very light
8	
9	Very light
10	
11	Fairly light
12	
13	Somewhat hard
14	
15	Hard
16	
17	Very hard
18	
19	Very, very hard
20	

Source: Adapted from G. V. Borg, "Psychological Basis of Perceived Exertion," *Medicine and Science in Sports and Exercise* 14 (1982): 377–81.

weight loss are not intensity but regularity, persistence, and duration. You will burn up almost the same number of calories walking at 3 mph for one hour as in running at 6 mph for half an hour. Focus on increasing the duration of your exercise, not on the intensity. As your body becomes more fit, the intensity at which you are exercising will naturally increase.

To achieve a high level of fitness, you need to exercise in your target zone for at least 20 to 30 minutes at least every other day. To burn calories, however, *any* extra physical activity will benefit you. While you may not lose very much weight by taking a leisurely stroll each day after dinner, you will at least be improving your lifestyle. And you may be able to eat slightly more than you would if you were watching TV after dinner instead of strolling.

Aerobic versus Anaerobic Exercise

The body burns energy in two major ways: with oxygen (aerobic), and without (anaerobic). The best way to burn calories consistently is to engage in *aerobic* activities. Aerobic exercise is the body's equivalent of a car cruising at a steady speed of 55 mph. It burns more gas than idling, but the engine is not straining. Aerobic activities include brisk walking, bicycling, swimming, dancing, aerobic exercises, or any rhythmic activity that elevates your heart rate for extended periods of time. These involve the continuous movement of large muscles and muscle groups. Aerobic exercises tend to raise the heart rate to your target zone or near it, and are excellent ways to burn calories and improve cardiovascular fitness and health.

Anaerobic exercise, on the other hand, occurs when you do the equivalent of flooring the accelerator of your car: the engine has to strain. In the body, the process exceeds our capacity to fuel the activity by the usual aerobic means. Anaerobic activities tend to be high intensity but are usually not sustained for very long. Racing up the stairs to answer the telephone, for example, is an anaerobic activity. Fuel is initially used without oxygen, and it usually leaves you feeling breathless or winded. This is a less efficient form of energy usage than aerobic exercise.

Weight lifting and other muscle-strengthening exercises are also anaerobic activities. While they contribute less to overall fitness, they are excellent ways to build muscle mass, and thus raise your energy usage (metabolic rate) while at rest. This is because muscles require more energy to sustain than fat and most other body tissues. The greater the size of your muscle mass, the more energy you will need to sustain your weight. A person with a lot of muscle mass can eat more than a person with a smaller muscle mass and not gain weight.

There is a paradoxical effect of doing a lot of muscle building, though. You may not see a decrease in weight initially. This is because as you replace fatty tissue with muscle tissue you are essentially replacing an oil-based substance (fat) with a water-based substance (muscle). As you know, fat floats on water, and the reason is that fat is lighter than water. You will often hear people say that muscle weighs more than fat. Fat takes up more space than muscle, however, so you will lose inches but not weight. Of course, if you are restricting your dietary intake of calories at the same time, you will lose weight, but the "trimming" may be more prominent than the scale changes. This is fine, since the numbers are not the point—it's how you feel (and look) that's important.

The Fitness Dimension of Your Personal Plan

You are now ready to design the fitness dimension of your Personal Plan. Your goal is to add the most physical activity to your week compatible with your schedule and physical health. In devising your fitness schedule and sticking to it, you must stay aware of two things.

First, exercise is a behavior. The kinds of behavior change you are aiming for are in many ways very similar to the kinds of lifestyle changes you have incorporated into the other areas of your plan, those covering diet and eating cues. That is, gradual change is more likely to become a permanent part of your lifestyle.

That leads us to the second point. You must make exercise a permanent part of your life. To be motivated to make these changes in physical activity, you can use the same tools discussed in Chapter 2. Review the short- and long-term benefits of successfully managing your weight, and recognize that they will likely last only when you incorporate additional physical activity into your lifestyle. (Note that it's okay, and sometimes even necessary, to skip exercising once in a while. If you have a commitment to physical activity, however, you'll soon get back into a regular routine.)

There are several steps to take in beginning your fitness program:

1. Get initial materials.
2. Choose some activities of daily living.
3. Choose some formal exercises tailored to your current level of physical fitness.
4. Set your schedule for frequency and duration.
5. Begin and end formal exercise sessions with warm-up and stretching activities.
6. Gradually build up the time or intensity—or both—of your activities.
7. Build up the variety of activities you engage in.
8. Keep going; work on maintenance.

1. Get initial materials. It's very easy to get the materials you need if you are starting out in the untrained, relatively unfit category, because you need little in the way of special equipment, just a pair of comfortable high-quality walking shoes, preferably with thick, flexible soles. Lycra and leotards aren't necessary. Wear loose clothes that are comfortable and stretchy. In cold weather, wear warm layers of loosely fitting clothes. In the summer months, wear lightweight and loose clothes to avoid overheating. If you are already relatively active, you may wish to consider purchasing equipment needed for specific exercises, such as a skiing machine, exercise bicycle, or treadmill, or equipment needed for specific sports such as golf or tennis. Even for the already physically active, though, it is not necessary to invest in special equipment; you are already equipped with a wonderful calorie-burning machine which can walk, jog, or run with low start-up costs—your legs and a good pair of shoes.

If you do wish to purchase exercise equipment, it is helpful to buy things you can use at home, regardless of the weather outside, and which you can use while doing other things like listening to music, watching television, or reading. Particularly for those with a weight problem, it is best to purchase high-quality new or used exercise equipment. Inexpensive models are not as likely to last and may become more costly in the long run. Since many people buy and never use exercise equipment, keep an eye on the classified ads for good quality equipment at bargain prices. Some useful equipment for aerobic exercise includes:

- Stationary bicycles. Look for a sturdy one with a comfortable seat, preferably whose handlebars also can move independently of the pedals, giving you a more extensive workout. Raise the seat high enough so that your legs are fully extended on the downstroke; this decreases knee strain. A rack for reading material is a useful option—as are devices that measure time, distance, and speed. This is a non-impact activity, so it is ideal for very overweight people.
- Cross-country skiing machines. These machines provide a good low-impact all-around aerobic workout. Again, look for durability. Using one of these machines requires a fair amount of coordination and balance, but it's a skill that can be mastered readily.
- Treadmills. Get one that is heavy duty, with a platform as long as possible, a handrail, and the ability to be inclined to simulate going uphill. Automatic shut-off is essential for motorized models. Good ones are expensive and take up a lot of space. Avoid cheap ones—they are no bargain in the long run. The non-motorized versions are less expensive but must be pushed along by you, which could strain your knees and hips.
- Stair-steppers. Look for one that is heavy duty, with variable tension. Unless they are equipped with special bars that simulate ski poles, stair-steppers exercise the legs only and may be difficult for people with balance problems.
- Rowers. Rowers can be hard on the back. Avoid pneumatic models; flywheel models are preferable. Learn proper rowing technique from an expert.
- Step aerobics (videotapes plus bench). These taped programs provide more intense exercise than non-step aerobic programs and can be obtained at a reasonable cost. Start with beginner-

level tapes and a 4-inch step. This form of exercise is good for the very overweight, fun, and a great confidence-builder.

Ideally you should choose things that are (or were in the past) enjoyable to you, as discussed in the assessment. And, as we stated in Chapter 2, a financial investment can often serve as a good motivator. Once you have the equipment you want, it's worth investing in a trip to a health club or a visit by a personal trainer so you can be taught proper exercise technique. This can both reduce the chance of injuries and improve results.

2. Choose your activities of daily living. There are two broad categories of activities: activities of daily living ("lifestyle" activities) and formal, programmed exercise or sports. For best results, incorporate both of these categories of activities into your Personal Plan of Action. Activities of daily living (sometimes abbreviated ADL) are in some ways easier to make part of your exercise routine than are sports or formal exercise. This is because they do not require setting aside a large block of time. They are an enhanced version of your usual physical activities and so do not have to be "scheduled," in the usual sense. You do have to get in the habit of expending more energy on a day-to-day basis, which is a behavior change, but you can continue to enhance your ADL no matter how busy you are or how busy you become.

There are two types of ADL: spontaneous activities (often called fidgeting), and what I call "throw-back" or lifestyle activities, doing things they way they used to be done before technology relieved us of the need to move our bodies.

The spontaneous activities are especially interesting because people seem to differ widely in the number of calories they burn up in unnecessary movement. This may be due to inherited differences in the nervous system, but it may also have a learned component. How many calories are we talking about? Studies have shown many extra calories a day can be burned up by very fidgety people. It should come as no surprise that most fidgeters are thin rather than obese.

How can you tell whether you are a person with a high or low level of spontaneous activity? You probably already know the answer to this question, but if you're not sure, table 7.4 provides a comparison for some typical activities.

While it is not clear whether you can become a fidgeter if you are not naturally inclined that way, it should be possible to consciously imitate some of the behaviors of fidgeters. If you are able to do this,

TABLE 7.4 WHAT'S YOUR LEVEL OF SPONTANEOUS ACTIVITY?

Situation	Non-Fidgeter	Fidgeter
Listening to music	Sits or lies still	Sits or stands, keeping beat
Standing in line	Stands still	Shifts weight frequently
Desk work—2 hours	No problem	Must get up regularly and stretch
Passing time at home	Watches TV or reads	Does something—tidies up, sews
Waiting for a train	Sits	Wanders around station
Relaxing	Sleeps, reads, watches TV	Takes a walk

you will burn additional calories without having to set aside any time for the effort. To increase your spontaneous physical activity level, it is probably best to focus on activities that seem a natural exaggeration of what you already do. For example, stand while talking on the phone instead of sitting or lying down. Make it a rule not to lie down except at night in bed. At home, do small tasks as soon as you think of them—don't store them up so you make only one trip downstairs, for instance.

In addition to spontaneous physical activity, there are a number of planned ways of increasing the number of calories you burn daily. These also take very little time out of your day and so don't need to be scheduled, the way exercise does. Think of these as "throw-backs" because they increase our physical work, counteracting the deleterious effects of the many labor-saving innovations of the past century.

The classic example of a throw-back activity is consciously decreasing your dependence on that great labor-saving device, the automobile. It is possible that a substantial contributor to the increase in obesity in this country is a decrease in walking. We are much less physically active than were previous generations of Americans.

While it is impractical for most of us to stop using the automobile, there are ways to reduce our reliance on cars and thereby increase our caloric expenditure. For example, is it possible to use public transportation to get to work? This not only helps the environment but burns calories, since you usually must walk a few blocks to get to and from the bus stop or train station. Side benefits include reduced stress (no driving in traffic) and the ability to catch up on reading or work while being transported. You can also get off one stop early, to work some extra walking into your day.

Other car-related ways to increase your day-to-day energy expenditure include walking or biking for nearby errands, or even just giving up the stress and time involved in searching for the closest parking spot by parking at the far end of the lot.

What are some other throw-back activities you can use to increase your calorie burning? Choose as many as you can from the following list. Add your own as they occur to you.

Use a carpet sweeper instead of the vacuum.
In the kitchen, avoid using electric appliances (chop and cut
    by hand).
Wash dishes in the sink and dry them with a towel.
Get up and change the channel instead of using the remote control.
Use a push mower instead of a self-propelled or riding mower.
Grow your own vegetables or plant a flower garden.
Take out the garbage.
Take the stairs instead of the elevator or escalator.

Making throw-back activities a natural part of your life can significantly increase the calories you burn without taking up a lot of time. Some will even save you money. It is probably easier for most inactive people to begin and stick with any of these activities of daily living for the long haul than it is to commit to a long-term plan of formal exercise. Take advantage of these activities by making them a part of your Personal Plan for fitness and weight management.

3. Choose formal exercises tailored to your fitness level. If you are relatively sedentary, it is probably best to begin with a progressive walking program, since this will provide you with a safe intensity of physical activity and still provide fitness and calorie-burning benefits. A walking program can grow with your growing level of fitness. Walking can lead to jogging or running, and can be done indoors (with a treadmill), at an enclosed public space (like a mall or an office complex), or outdoors. Walking can be a social activity, done with friends or family, or enjoyed alone as a time to think and relax. I'll use walking as an example in later sections to discuss how to schedule your formal exercise periods, how to use warm-up and cool-down exercises, and how to progressively increase the frequency, duration, and intensity of your exercise sessions.

Even if you have already been exercising regularly and are at least moderately fit, a progressive walking program can provide a good aerobic workout and can be a part of your fitness plan. If you are in this already-fit category and have no medical problems that limit your activities, your choice of sports and exercises can be much broader right from the start.

Again, your choice of activities is best made keeping in mind the assessment you completed earlier in this chapter. Choose activities you enjoy or enjoyed when you were younger or more fit. A list of some of the most popular aerobic activities (in addition to brisk walking) follows. Please check off at least two that you are interested in trying. They are listed roughly in increasing order of difficulty, in terms of intensity of exercise and ease of learning and doing them. A brief discussion of each one follows this list.

Common Sports and Exercises

Low-impact aerobics _____

Cycling/stationary bicycling _____

Swimming/water aerobics _____

Golf (without cart) _____

Rollerskating/rollerblading _____

Team sports _____

Step aerobics and aerobic dancing _____

Jogging/running/treadmil _____

Rowing _____

Cross-country skiing/machine _____

Squash/racquetball/tennis _____

Low-impact aerobics are easy to do because a variety of videos are available and no equipment is required. These exercises can be done at home anytime you choose, or you can join a class at a local YMCA or recreation center (classes have the added benefit of camaraderie). Choose an aerobic routine that is designed for someone at your current fitness level. Be sure to check your pulse periodically, such as after a set of exercises (stop the videotape). If you are at your target heart rate, good. If you are well below it, you can either do the described exercises more vigorously or get a videotape for more advanced exercisers. If you are above your target zone, just march in place until your heart rate slows to the target zone or your comfort zone on the perceived exertion scale. Remember, you do not always have to follow every movement in the video. Pace yourself! You can either try another videotape for beginners, or do the recommended exercises less vigorously or for fewer repetitions than suggested.

If you use *a stationary bike,* you don't even have to know how to ride a two-wheeler. If you know how to ride a *bicycle,* the advantage of cycling outdoors is the change of scenery and fresh air. Be sure to wear a helmet for safety. Be careful not to simply glide without turning the pedals or your workout will be no more vigorous than a leisurely stroll. If you are very unfit or have a problem with balance, the indoor variety provides the same workout with greater safety and can be done in all kinds of weather. Outdoor cyclers can benefit from having a stationary bicycle for inclement weather. I prefer the kind of bike with "dual action," so you can work out with your arms, legs, or both. To avoid knee problems, make sure you set the seat height properly. By adapting the suggestions in section 6 (below) on building the intensity of a walking program, you can make your cycling grow more challenging as your fitness increases.

Swimming and water aerobics (*aqua-aerobics*) are superb aerobic exercises and especially useful for very overweight people who will benefit from the feeling of buoyancy the water provides. Because they are low impact, aqua-aerobics are also good for people with joint problems or low back problems. Like cycling, the intensity of the exercise can be tailored to your level of fitness. Again, aim for your target heart rate. A problem with swimming is that your activity may tend to end as cold weather approaches. Plan ahead: join an indoor pool or replace swimming in the winter months with some other activity to help avoid weight gain.

Golf is an excellent low-impact aerobic exercise if you do it right. It needs to be done regularly to obtain the maximum benefit. Also, no golf carts or wheeled carriers allowed! Golf provides lots of brisk walking; cost and seasonality are the major drawbacks. Check out public facilities for price breaks.

Rollerskating/blading have seen renewed popularity of late. For safety, be sure to wear protective gear. It can be done near home, or at a park. It requires excellent balance and some learning. For indoor exercise during cold weather, consider a roller rink or indoor ice rink.

If you noted during your assessment that you used to enjoy participating in *team sports,* this category may still be an option. There are a surprising variety of team activities in most neighborhoods. Check with local high schools, employee groups, religious organizations, and men's and women's clubs, and scan the local newspapers as well as postings on community and grocery store bulletin boards. You may even be able to start your own team with friends, or organize games at gatherings of family or friends.

Step aerobics. This aerobic activity differs from and is often more intensive than non-step aerobics. It is also low impact, and many people find it easier to follow. The only equipment is a specially designed bench or step made of heavy plastic, and high-quality footwear designed for aerobics. Step aerobics is good as an indoor and bad weather activity that can burn more calories generally than non-step aerobics or aerobic dancing. There are many excellent videotapes available for home exercisers. Step aerobic classes have the disadvantage of scheduling and travel to and from them, but the advantage of camaraderie.

Jogging, running, and using a treadmill are more intensive forms of walking. As discussed, in terms of calorie burning there is little difference between walking an hour at 2½ mph or jogging a half-hour at 5 mph. However, the intensity of the activity is much higher, and you will build better cardiovascular fitness and endurance at the faster pace. Take care, though, and do not pursue these more intensive forms of aerobic activity until you are able to do so comfortably. If jogging gets your heart rate above your target rate, you should not jog until you have increased your fitness through a progressive walking/jogging program to a level where jogging alone no longer results in a pulse faster than your target. These more rapid paces are also higher impact than walking, and are more likely to result in injuries. It is best to give yourself at least one or two days off per week. An excellent schedule for jogging or running is every other day. Treadmills enable you to continue the activity in inclement weather, at home. Again, footwear designed especially for jogging will help to minimize the risk of overuse injuries.

Rowing can be done as a team sport, alone *al fresco,* or using a machine equivalent. The machine reproduces the exercise nicely, but you don't get the same scenery. This form of exercise may be hard on the back if not done properly; rowing technique is best learned from a professional. Check with local crew teams for clinics or private instruction in proper technique. About 60 percent of the work of rowing is done by the legs when performed properly.

Cross-country skiing is an excellent total body aerobic exercise. It's most enjoyable on snow, but high-quality ski machines provide the same workout and high calorie burning. This activity requires a fair amount of coordination and balance and is not ideal for the unfit beginner.

Squash, racquetball, and tennis provide a competitive workout; because they are usually high-intensity, high-impact activities, injuries and joint strain are not uncommon. They're great exercise if you do them regularly and are already physically fit, but they're not recommended for the unfit or weekend exerciser as a way to burn calories or become fit. You need to have a regular partner who plays at your level. Racquet sports are neither good exercise nor much fun if your opponent plays at a significantly different level than you do.

This list of activities provides just some examples of the many options available. You can assess other activities, too, and determine whether they are appropriate for you. Determine whether the activity is high or low impact, whether the intensity level is right for you, whether it is competitive or noncompetitive, individual or team or group, and whether you are likely to enjoy it and be willing to employ the activity as a regular part of your fitness program throughout the year. It is best to avoid the latest fad exercises or sports, especially if they require a substantial investment in equipment or training.

Ideally, you have now decided on a couple of activities from the above list to add to your fitness plan. If you are starting out at a low level of fitness, you are better off starting with a progressive walking program, adding the more vigorous activities as your fitness improves.

4. Set your schedule. As you know, sticking to a regular program of physical activities can be crucial to your long-term success at weight management. To consistently sustain a level of physical activity above your current level, it is helpful to devise a schedule you can live with. Just as things get done more reliably at work when a time is set aside for them, your fitness plan will become a reality only if you set aside the needed time.

How much time is needed? To achieve a higher level of physical fitness and burn a significant number of calories, plan to spend 20 to 30 minutes at your target heart rate at least every other day. If you throw in 5 minutes to stretch and warm up, and 5 minutes to cool down, this is a minimum of 30 minutes per session. If the activity is done at home or at work, no travel time need be added. If you must travel—to a health club, for example—figure in travel time and time for changing clothes.

Regardless of how busy you are, it should be possible to schedule this amount of time if you make the commitment to do so. Many people have successfully utilized part of their lunchtime at work. Others are freshest in the morning and prefer scheduling activities early in the morning. Still others prefer early evening during the week. On weekends, it is often best to choose a time early in the day so as not to interfere with other activities, or have other activities interfere with your exercise.

Many people find it easier to keep up their exercise regimen if they keep a written record. Write down what days and times you have set aside for exercise to serve as a reminder of your commitment. You can use a card or a schedule book; keep the card or book with you, or post it with a magnet in the kitchen. You will be tempted to break this commitment when you are busy or tired, but remember, this commitment is just as important as anything else in your schedule. Dr. George Sheehan once said, "Not all my workouts have been good ones, but I have never finished a workout feeling worse than when I started."

Another technique that helps people stick to a schedule is keeping a checklist on your schedule card, or on a separate summary log. You can then check off the times when you have completed each session. Use photocopies of the Log of Physical Activities (page 198). (The kilocalories expended take into account the person's weight.) A completed sample log is shown on page 199.

By keeping a record, you will have a written reminder that you have kept to your commitment or, if you need to skip an activity session, you'll know that you have fallen short of your scheduled goal. This way, you will be more likely to make up for any shortfall in exercise than if you relied on an unwritten schedule, or no schedule at all. It is extraordinarily easy for other things to intrude on your scheduled fitness time unless you keep track of it and commit to making up for lost time.

One problem many people have with scheduled fitness activities is that during the preparation and action stages of their Personal Plan, they may be overly ambitious in their scheduling of physical activities, perhaps in number of sessions, intensity of exercise, or duration of each session. It may seem as if more should be better, and if that's the case, why not take advantage of your peak motivational state?

If you keep the long-term goal of weight maintenance in mind, you can see how an overly aggressive exercise schedule can have a negative rather than a positive effect. You may indeed stick to a grueling, time-consuming schedule initially, but after a while you probably won't be able to keep it up. Then, the level you are able to maintain will likely lead to weight regain rather than maintenance. Also, once you have accomplished your weight goal, the grueling schedule will

LOG OF PHYSICAL ACTIVITIES

Date	Scheduled Activity	Completed Activity How Long/Far	Kilocalories Expended

seem excessive and unnecessary. There is a tendency to stop doing these activities almost entirely, yet we know that regular exercise at a moderate level is necessary for giving you the best chance at keeping your weight stable.

To avoid this problem, it is best to pick a moderate and sustainable amount of time to commit to fitness activities from the start. It will be much easier to continue a level of activity that fits comfortably into your schedule than a more aggressive level that requires putting other commitments aside.

5. Use warm-up, stretching, and cool-down procedures. Injuries are more likely to occur when you fail to get your body gradually ready for exercise, and exercise-related injuries provide a sure-fire excuse for abandoning your Personal Plan. Once you have lost your initial momentum, it can be extremely difficult to get going again. To avoid these interruptions, warm-ups and cool-downs are essential.

For a walking program, an appropriate warm-up is to walk more slowly than your usual exercise pace for a few minutes, then gradually pick up the pace. You should also do some stretching exercises, such as the following (two or three repetitions of each).

Floor touch:
> With your knees only slightly bent, move your upper body toward the ground, touching it with the palms of your hands, bending at the waist. Now hold that position without bouncing for the count of ten, and slowly stand up. If your lower back

LOG OF PHYSICAL ACTIVITIES (EXAMPLE)

Date	Scheduled Activity	Completed Activity How Long/Far	Kilocalories Expended
Mon, April 2	Walking	30 minutes	200
Tues, April 3	—		
Wed, April 4	Walking	40 minutes	267
Thurs, April 5	—		
Fri, April 6	Walking	30 minutes	200
Sat, April 7	Exercise bicycle	25 minutes	175
Sun, April 8	Walking	45 minutes	300

Total time spent during the week: 170 minutes (2 hrs 50 min)
Total kilocalories expended: 1142

sometimes hurts, you can reduce the strain on it by doing this exercise with your legs crossed instead of parallel.

Toe touch:
   With your right leg held straight out on the seat of a chair or bench, and your left leg straight and on the ground, lean forward and touch the toes of your right foot. Again, do not bounce your body. You should feel the stretch in the hamstring muscles at the back of the thigh. Now switch legs.

Wall push:
   Stand about three or four feet away from a wall. Now lean forward while pushing against the wall with your hands, keeping your feet flat on the ground. Hold this stretched position for the count of ten, then stand up straight.

These warm-ups can be adapted for most exercises and sports. For instance, if you are cycling instead of walking, start by doing stretching exercises, then cycle slowly for the first few minutes to ease into your cycling workout.

At the end of your exercise session, it is best to cool down slowly, giving your body a chance to adjust gradually to less activity. You should not be exercising so vigorously that you need to lie down, panting at the end of the session. To cool down, perform the same activity you were doing at a slow pace for a few minutes. For instance, if you were jogging, walk. If you were cycling at 10 mph, cycle at 5 mph. If you were playing tennis, walk. Stretching exercises should also be used at the end of your cool-down period.

6. Build up the time or intensity of your activity. If you start an exercise program and are doing it the same way for half an hour every other day, you will soon notice that it seems to take less and less effort as the weeks go on. Your aerobic endurance is increasing. Your body is becoming more fit! Your heart rate will also begin to dip below your target rate at the same level of intensity that used to make it strain.

When this happens, you may also get bored with the lack of challenge. You can even become so efficient at the activity that you burn fewer calories to complete the session. Since our aim is to increase fitness and burn calories, it is clear that you must increase the time or intensity (or both) of the activity as time goes on.

Whether you increase the time you spend exercising, the intensity of your workout, or both will affect the benefits you receive. If you only increase the time but not the intensity you will increase the calories burned approximately in proportion to the increase in time spent. A half hour of walking at 3 mph burns about 160 calories (for a 150-pound person). An hour burns about 320 calories. For weight control purposes this is all we really care about.

For fitness purposes, however, walking at 2 mph will not increase your fitness to a very high level, no matter how long you walk. But increasing the intensity of the activity (walking 3 mph while swinging your arms, for example) will increase both the number of calories burned and your fitness level. Gradually increasing the intensity will also keep you exercising at the appropriate target heart rate for your level of fitness. By focusing on working at a moderate to high level of intensity you will gradually increase your workout intensity as fitness improves.

Increasing both the duration and the intensity of your exercise will yield the maximum benefits in both calories burned and fitness. The disadvantage is that such an exercise program may be too aggressive for many people, and it can increase the risk of injuries and burnout. Unless you are an athlete training for a competitive event, there is no need to push yourself to the edge of your physical limits, and there is potential danger in doing so. Keep it low-key and enjoyable.

Thus, for the initially not-particularly-fit person trying to lose weight and maintain the loss, it is probably best to increase just the duration but not the intensity of the exercise regimen at first. Once you have reached an exercise duration of about 30 to 45 minutes and

TABLE 7.5 PROGRESSIVE WALKING PROGRAM FOR BEGINNERS

Week	Frequency	Time Walking at Target Rate	Warm-up/ Stretching/ Cool Down (5 minutes each)	Total Exercise Time
1	3–5 × per wk	5 minutes	10 minutes	15 minutes
2	3–5 × per wk	7 minutes	10 minutes	17 minutes
3	3–5 × per wk	10 minutes	10 minutes	20 minutes
4	3–5 × per wk	12 minutes	10 minutes	22 minutes
5	3–5 × per wk	15 minutes	10 minutes	25 minutes
6	3–5 × per wk	17 minutes	10 minutes	27 minutes
7	3–5 × per wk	20 minutes	10 minutes	30 minutes
8	3–5 × per wk	22 minutes	10 minutes	32 minutes
9	3–5 × per wk	25 minutes	10 minutes	35 minutes
10	3–5 × per wk	30 minutes	10 minutes	40 minutes
11	3–5 × per wk	30 minutes	10 minutes	40 minutes
12 and beyond	3–5 × per wk	30 minutes	10 minutes	40 minutes

your fitness has improved, then you may want to gradually increase the intensity of the activity, keeping the time fixed. These suggestions are incorporated in the sample progressive walking program shown in table 7.5. Keep in mind that you must monitor your exercise intensity so that you walk at a speed that puts you at your target heart rate, or your target perceived exertion.

Beginning at week 12, begin very slowly quickening your pace if you can stay close to your target heart rate. When and if reaching your initial target heart rate becomes too easy for you, try stepping up to the next target rate category (see table 7.2, "Calculating Your Target Heart Rate"). You may need to switch from a brisk walk to a jog at some point along this sequence. Do not advance to the next week until you are comfortable completing the current week's walking.

A similar progression can be used for virtually any other physical activity you choose to incorporate into your fitness plan.

7. Build up the variety of your activities. While a progressive walking program is an excellent way to burn calories and increase fitness, you may get bored with only a single activity. This does not mean that you should stop walking and replace walking with another form of exercise. It is better to continue walking, perhaps at a slightly reduced duration if you have time constraints, and add something new. Athletes call this *cross-training*. Cross-training can reduce the risk of injuries as well as add variety to your workout. Don't reduce the walking time until you have reached at least the tenth week of the progressive plan described above—after you have attained some mastery of the activity. In this way, you can have a sense of accomplishment and satisfaction, which makes it more likely that you will want to add other activities to your fitness plan.

What should you add if you started off with increasing your activities of daily living and a progressive walking program? Use your assessment as a guide to the kinds of activities you may enjoy, or add something from the list of formal activities discussed in this chapter. An added advantage of team or group activities is that meeting new people will help keep you motivated, and will expand your athletic interests and capabilities.

8. Keep going—maintenance. As with the other aspects of your Personal Plan of Action, your fitness program is beneficial only if it becomes part of your life from now on. The next chapter will focus exclusively on the problem of maintaining positive behavior changes, including self-monitoring, paying attention to changing conditions, and learning problem-solving skills.

Here are a number of tactics, from the general to the specific, which can help you adhere to a fitness program.

- Start off slowly, and build gradually to attainable goals. There is nothing more likely to lead to quitting a fitness program than unrealistic goals, including an excessive time commitment or an excessively intensive exercise level. The latter, of course, can even be dangerous. Gradually increasing your activities will be satisfying and will give you a well-earned sense of accomplishment.
- Pick activities that you enjoy. You may have to work up to these activities gradually if you have not been physically active for a while. Persisting in a progressive walking program will pay off as pre-training for more vigorous activities. Remember the payoff. Don't think of your fitness plan as a dreaded chore. Focus on the activities you can see yourself enjoying, and give yourself a chance to appreciate that you are indeed accomplishing something. Notice how you feel more fit, don't get tired as

easily, and gain all of the other benefits of increasing physical activity described at the beginning of this chapter.

- Watch small children and follow their lead in being naturally active and loving to move. Go out with them in the evening when they ride their bikes, play catch in the sideyard, spend family time being active. If you don't have small children, you might play with the neighbors' children or your relatives' children. Invite the parents to join in.

- Find a role model or a fitness buddy. A role model should be someone whose circumstances are similar to yours but who manages to stay active and fit. If possible, make your role model your fitness partner. If not, identify a friend or relative who is also interested in becoming more fit or losing weight and enlist his or her support and participation. You are far less likely to skip an exercise session when you have someone you exercise with or someone who is waiting to exercise with you.

- Set small, realistic goals. You can get tremendous benefits just by walking. You don't need to begin a walking program telling yourself that you next need to move to running if you are going to be successful.

- Make moving, rather than exercise, the goal. How can I get my body moving? By walking instead of taking the escalator. Or walking on the escalator, if you have to take the escalator.

- Keep a schedule and exercise log. The old Chinese adage holds true: "The palest ink is better than the best memory." This tip was discussed earlier but is worth repeating. Make yourself aware of your commitment to fitness, and track your progress. It is also satisfying to see your abilities increase on paper, since progress is often slow but steady. The log serves as a reminder of how your fitness is increasing through your efforts. Again, writing your workouts into your weekly calendar will help to increase the likelihood of your remaining active.

- Plan ahead for difficulties. Recognize that most people stop exercising during an illness. There is a natural tendency to let the program slip after you have appropriately missed some exercise when recovering from an illness. When you're derailed, recognize how important it is to *plan* how you'll get moving again. The same thing holds for holidays and vacations. Make a firm plan and commit to how you will resume your exercise program *before* you begin the celebration or leave town to visit friends or relatives. Then stick to the plan.

- Recognize the two or three most common excuses you give yourself for not exercising, and then develop an appropriate response. Talk back to yourself the way a good friend would talk to you! Write these responses down and keep them handy. Review them regularly.
- Set things out the night before. To avoid rushing around at the last minute gathering your things, set equipment or clothing for exercising out the night before, by the door, or in your car so you will see them on your way to work or upon arriving home. Nothing will deter you from exercising more than if you are always late for work because you can't find your walking shoes.
- Make it interesting. In addition to adding variety to your program, you can change the scenery (walk a different route), carry a portable radio, cassette player, or CD player, or exercise while reading or watching TV. If you are someone who enjoys clothes, buy attractive, comfortable exercise clothes. And enjoy watching them become looser!
- Look for new ways to be active. Try a new activity. Invest time in finding and maintaining exercise activities that you enjoy. Don't just decide you need to take an exercise class and then join the most convenient one. Find out about the music, the instructor, the setting, and so on. Observe the class and talk to the instructor *before* you take the class. That way the instructor knows you and has a vested interest in your enjoying the class.
- Give yourself rewards. While fitness is its own reward, a little something extra won't hurt, especially if it's something related to your new fitness. Time for yourself is an excellent reward.
- Become a knowledgeable exerciser. Developing an intellectual interest in fitness and different sports and activities can help maintain your enthusiasm. Subscribe to fitness magazines, join local teams or interest groups, and see your fitness program become a very satisfying and integral part of your life.

Remember, to be losing, you have to keep moving!

EIGHT

Keeping It Off

The most difficult struggle for many people who have lost weight is not the initial battle but its aftermath. How can victory be maintained in the period following the weight loss? Why, when it entails *less* deprivation, is maintenance often harder than weight loss?

The reasons vary from person to person, but frequently regaining lost weight is the result of the way the person approached weight loss in the first place. In an "all-or-nothing" approach, the person diets with a bang—eating nothing at all except water or diet sodas. Or the person may find an aggressive diet that touts the value of a single food or food group, such as fruits, vegetables, high-fiber foods, protein, complex carbohydrates, even ice cream. The person may religiously follow that diet for a week, even a month. Others may start an intensive exercise program that takes hours of time each day, along with a restricted diet.

Do people lose weight on such diets? You bet! The trouble is, such diets are of no value in keeping weight off for the long haul. This is because they cannot be followed indefinitely. They do not address the causes of the person's weight problem, and they teach the person nothing about how to manage weight down the road. Because the person is either "on" the diet or "not on" the diet, there is nothing in between, no maintenance plan. That's why we call this "all-or-nothing" behavior.

Many people, unfortunately, find "all-or-nothing" approaches irresistible. They are used to not dealing effectively with a problem until it becomes intolerable, then seeking a rapid cure. This approach can lead to yo-yo dieting. Even if it has no ill effects on your health (the scientific verdict is still out), yo-yo dieting is at the least ineffective. And it's discouraging for anyone to face repeated episodes of dieting and weight regain.

Having read this book, you now know about a far better approach than all-or-nothing behavior. You have developed a Personal Plan of Action for weight management which was designed *by you* after careful assessment of your individual strengths and needs. It contains not just a "diet," but also a plan for healthful eating after the weight loss, a plan for behavior change, and a fitness plan. You have looked closely at your reasons for wanting to lose weight and maintain a healthful weight. You know what motivates you best and longest. You know the stages of change, and you are ready.

The fact is that, throughout this book, you have been methodically building the foundation for maintaining your weight loss. In each chapter you learned a specific technique for maintaining the progress you make during the action stage of your Personal Plan. You know what lifestyle changes are necessary for you to succeed.

The purpose of this chapter is to reinforce some of the important ingredients of long-term weight management. We will study the characteristics of people who are most successful at losing weight and keeping it off, and compare them with people who are the least successful. We will then summarize how you can put yourself squarely into the "most successful" camp. Let's begin by looking at the results of some recent research studies.

Successful Maintainers: What Do We Know?

First, the bad news. Most research studies in the past have shown relatively poor long-term maintenance of lost weight a few years or more after a weight loss program. This includes programs that emphasize behavior modification as well as programs that emphasize aggressive dieting such as very-low-calorie, liquid protein diets. Fewer than one out of ten people in these studies succeeded in maintaining a substantial weight loss in the long run.

Before you get discouraged, however, let me say that these studies do not tell the whole story. There have been some studies that show a considerably better result among people *not* enrolled in formal research studies. How can this be? Probably because people who lose weight on their own, perhaps with the help of friends and information they learn from personal experience and books, are different from the average research "subject." They may not have as severe a problem, or may be less likely to have associated problems, like depression, which interfere with successful weight management.

Research studies also suggest that having continual contact with others in the weight loss program is an important part of weight maintenance. When a program ends abruptly, the results are poor. With ongoing support, perhaps as infrequently as every two weeks or even less often than that, maintenance of weight loss is much improved. In a self-help program such as your Personal Plan, there has never been any one-on-one contact between the program and the participant. Does this mean that the benefit of personal contact would not apply in this situation? I believe it does apply, and that ongoing contact would be beneficial even to people who have developed a Personal Plan.

You can secure the additional "maintenance insurance" that regular ongoing contact provides in one of two ways. You can join or form your own support group for people who have recently lost weight and are trying to maintain the loss. Or, you can develop a support system for yourself which provides some of the same benefits as a support group. In Chapter 4 you read about the key ingredients of a good maintenance system. The ingredients of this system which relate most directly to the concept of ongoing contact are the following:

1. Learning to talk positively to yourself. Being your own cheerleader can keep you going.
2. Keeping records. Self-monitoring of food, exercise, and behavior is like discussing your progress with someone else.
3. Continuing your buddy system. Keep in touch with your dieting partner during the maintenance stage.
4. Consulting your written lists of substitute activities and problem-solving actions when old eating behaviors or situations threaten.

Although in a Personal Plan of Action you will not have the benefit of ongoing contact through a therapist or in a group setting (unless you choose to seek one out), you can obtain much of the benefit by nurturing your own contacts, through both your people-support system and such tools as talking to yourself in a positive way, keeping written lists of useful behaviors, and self-monitoring activities.

What do studies show about the characteristics of successful maintainers compared to regainers? There are only a handful of studies in this area, but the themes are similar to a 1990 study by Dr. Susan Kayman and others at UCLA. They compared the behaviors of a group of 30 women who had successfully lost 20 percent or more of their initial weight and maintained the loss at least two years, to 44 women who had regained their lost weight, and 34 "controls" who had not lost any weight. Their findings included the following information that can be useful to us:

1. The successful maintainers were much more likely (73%) than the relapsers (39%) to have lost weight by devising a personal eating plan after making the decision to lose weight.
2. The maintainers were more than twice as likely (76%) than the relapsers (36%) to have exercised regularly to help lose weight.
3. The relapsers were far more likely (47%) than the maintainers (3%) to have used appetite-suppressing pills to lose weight.
4. While 72 per cent of the relapsers attended weight loss programs and groups, only 10 percent of the maintainers attended such groups. Ninety percent of the maintainers achieved long-term weight loss on their own.
5. The maintainers, unlike the relapsers, were aware that they needed to continue to be conscious of their eating and physical activity behaviors.
6. Ninety percent of maintainers were still exercising regularly after their weight loss (at least 3 times per week, 30 minutes per session), while only 34 percent of the regainers did so. Even those regainers who did exercise regularly did so less frequently and less vigorously than the maintainers.
7. Regainers ate 4.6 snacks per day, while maintainers ate only 1.5 snacks on a typical day. Regainers also ate more candies and chocolate and were more likely to skip breakfast than maintainers and controls.
8. While women in all the groups reported having stress or troubling issues in their lives, they coped in different ways. Few of the regainers (10%) used problem solving or confrontational ways of coping, compared to 95% of the maintainers and 60% of the average-weight controls.
9. Many regainers (70%) reported dealing with problems by "escape-avoidance," such as eating, sleeping, drinking, smoking, taking tranquilizers, or simply wishing the problem would go away. Fewer than half as many maintainers (33%) coped in these ineffective ways.
10. While 70% of maintainers reported seeking outside support in dealing with problems, either by talking out their feelings or seeking professional help, only 38% of regainers did these things.

The results of the above study bring to light a number of lessons that may be useful to you in thinking about your strategies for maintaining weight loss.

Most, if not all, of the habits of successful maintainers can be learned, even if they are not already a part of your repertoire. Does emulating the behavior pattern of successful maintainers guarantee that you, too, will be successful? Unfortunately, no. But it is likely that your chances will be vastly improved. Having a clear plan of action is just as critical to weight maintenance as it is to weight loss, and your Personal Plan, with few modifications, can serve you well after the action phase of active weight loss is complete.

Weight maintenance after weight loss uses the same strategies as the weight loss phase. That is, it is still important to pay attention to the reasons why you chose to lose weight. They are still applicable even though you may have already lost the weight you set out to lose. It is particularly important to remind yourself of the benefits you are enjoying since losing weight, and not to forget what your life was like before developing and following your Personal Plan.

Regarding the goals of maintenance, there are many similarities to the goals of the weight loss phase. The goal of maintenance must be reasonable. That is, you should not expect to stay within a pound of your lowest weight. Instead, recognize that weight management means managing your weight within a reasonable *range*. This may be a 5-pound or 10-pound range for some, or as much as 20 pounds for those who were obese.

While it is important in maintenance to keep close tabs on your weight, you should recognize that your weight may vary by as much as several pounds from day to day. This is largely due to changes in the body's state of hydration—how much water you are carrying in your tissues. Increases in body water are sometimes hormonally driven. Many premenopausal women especially notice fluid retention during the days right before menstruating. For other people, eating foods high in salt may result in fluid retention. Thus, it is possible to eat the same number of calories yet gain water weight during some periods.

Within this variation, however, it is a good idea to keep close watch on your weight and on how your clothes fit. An increase above the goal range you have achieved or a snugly fitting outfit may signal a maintenance problem. Many successful maintainers weigh themselves daily (weighing yourself more than once a day yields no further information). The idea is not to focus exclusively on the number of pounds, though, since the pounds are an imperfect reflection of what is really being managed during maintenance—your behavior.

During maintenance, the best way to evaluate your behavior is through self-monitoring of as many items as you can manage. The more you monitor, the better—within limits. At a minimum you should monitor your weight, your food portions (or fat grams), and your physical activity, using the forms in Chapters 6 and 7. For those whose Personal Plan reflected a need to control inappropriate eating cues, ongoing monitoring of eating situations and what you did to deal with them is critical. All this monitoring should take less than 15 minutes per day. This is a reasonable investment of time for maintaining your hard-won success. Try to stay aware of the pleasures of maintaining a healthful weight, as opposed to the pleasures of food. For instance, cancel your subscription to a gourmet food magazine and replace it with a subscription to a fitness magazine. Take pride in your fitness, positive health attitudes, and appearance.

Maintenance Pitfalls

Despite the best of intentions, you must recognize that there will be lapses and even relapses along the path, but we hope you will not suffer total collapse. What do these terms mean? A lapse can be described as a slip from desired behaviors. An example is eating the second piece of chocolate cake when you were not hungry. Lapses are very common and no cause for alarm. I am often more concerned about people who suffer no lapses than those who have frequent lapses. Lapses are, by definition, temporary. When the cake is gone, the lapse is over. It does not spell the end of your Personal Plan. You must simply move on, record the event dutifully as part of your monitoring, and learn something from it, whether it is how to avoid the situation, how to substitute another behavior, or simply how to compensate for the lapse in some other way over the next day. No lapses means no practice in dealing with situations that need more work. No lapses may lead to or reflect all-or-nothing thinking.

A relapse, on the other hand, is when you stop adhering to your Personal Plan in ongoing, major ways. Relapse may occur early, or at any time during maintenance. Often relapse happens when you stop self-monitoring. The needed vigilance to avoid weight regain may seem too big a burden, or you may simply become confident in your ability to manage your weight with less control. Unfortunately, this doesn't usually turn out to be the case.

If rebellion or lack of interest in weight management is the problem, it can help to refocus yourself. Recall your work in Chapters 1 and 2, "Why Lose Weight?" and "Getting Ready" and see whether your situation or feelings have changed. If they have not, this rethinking of your Personal Plan may help re-invigorate your motivation. If overconfidence is the problem, sometimes only a trial of less vigilance was needed. Perhaps you have learned enough so that less stringent control is needed, but perhaps not—and in that case you will see that you cannot relax the requirements of your Personal Plan but must learn to accept the ongoing necessity of adhering to it.

When all else fails, and it is clear that a relapse has occurred, do not lose faith in yourself. It is discouraging to relapse, but you must recognize that multiple efforts are usually required to permanently change ingrained behavior patterns, especially eating patterns that are reinforced by our environment and our culture. The average cigarette smoker trying to quit makes several attempts before success, and even then may relapse years later. Changing eating habits is, in many ways, more difficult. You can't simply quit eating. You should expect that it may take more than one try to get it right. You will learn something from each attempt, particularly if you are working from a Personal Plan that provides insights into the why's of your behavior. Positive self-talk is important in dealing with a relapse. The bottom line for relapsers is that you can pick yourself up and try again, wiser for the effort.

A collapse, however, is something entirely different. A collapse is a relapse accompanied by a loss of interest in change. At times the person in collapse may feel hopeless, and may be depressed. When a collapse occurs or threatens, it is often advisable to seek professional help from a physician, counselor, or therapist experienced in helping people with weight problems. The solution may be to choose a different "reasonable" goal, perhaps to stabilize at the current weight instead of trying to lose weight again.

When you do experience a lapse or relapse, it is helpful to apply the problem-solving approach favored by most successful maintainers—objective and specific identification of the problem. For example, "eating when X happens" is easier to solve than the nonspecific problem of "overeating." If you suspect there are inappropriate eating situations causing your relapse but are unsure of what they are, you can resurrect the "watch trick" described in Chapter 5. If you think overall food quantity or dietary fat percentage is the problem, you can begin a period of "super analyst" dietary monitoring to get a better handle on where you are going wrong.

Problem Solving for Successful Maintenance

Whatever you do, do not allow yourself to deal with (or rather *not* deal with) problems by escape-avoidance behaviors such as more eating, smoking, pills, or wishful thinking (as in "Maybe the problem will solve itself"). This is maladaptive, self-defeating behavior that could negate everything you have accomplished.

Once you have identified one or more specific problem areas, the next step in the problem-solving approach is brainstorming to come up with a number of possible solutions. The point of brainstorming is not to arrive brilliantly at the fail-proof solution, but to give yourself some ideas to try out, the more the better. Not all the brainstormed solutions need to be good ones. It can even be helpful to think of a few ridiculous ones, to give yourself a good, healthy laugh. (For example, have you considered heating all your silverware to 300° before dinner?)

Then, armed with alternative behaviors, choose one or more that you think have the best chance of working. It's not as important to be correct initially in your choice of a solution as it is just to try something. Look at this as a little experiment, knowing that the worst you are likely to do is not help the situation. You will learn something from the experiment regardless of its outcome.

The last step in the problem-solving approach, of course, is to try out your proposed solution or solutions, keeping in mind that you may need to fine-tune your solution, or try another one entirely. Even if you cannot entirely resolve the problem, it is a good bet that the problem-solving approach will result in some improvement. At the same time, it will give you the confidence and pleasure that come from constructively addressing your problems instead of hiding from them.

Support for Your Maintenance Phase

One important strategy used by maintainers to help solve problems is having a network of friends and relatives to turn to. The related concept of a buddy system was described as a key ingredient of weight loss in Chapter 4. It is equally useful during the maintenance phase.

Being able to discuss problems with others has many advantages. Getting encouragement from others can make you feel the problem is not all that bad. Discussion will also help you crystallize the issues and create viable solutions; it will enable you to test the likely response to your solutions; and, finally, it will give you immediate positive feedback regarding the problem and your ability to solve it.

Maintaining Healthy Habits

The various tools described during the development of your Personal Plan were presented as assessment or weight loss devices, but they are equally useful as maintenance tools. They include: stimulus-control devices, such as keeping tempting foods out of the house or out of sight; eating only in one room of the house; changing to a low-fat, higher volume diet with increased emphasis on foods lower on the food guide pyramid; and adding spices instead of fats to improve the taste of foods. Changes in eating habits are maintenance tools, too. They include teaching yourself to eat more slowly, in smaller bites, on smaller plates, in regular meals, taken only when you are physically hungry. And, calorie-burning devices such as increasing incidental activities and spontaneous activities, in addition to formal exercise, will help you successfully maintain your weight loss.

To keep these tools fresh, you may find it helpful during maintenance to vary your emphasis from time to time. For example, you may engage in a different form of monitoring from month to month, setting aside February and March, for instance, for exercise monitoring, since it is a time when cold weather makes getting enough physical activity more problematic, and April and May for monitoring your fat intake as warm weather approaches. Similarly, you can vary the forms of physical activity you emphasize from season to season, or vary the kinds of foods you use to fill your pyramid boxes based on the seasonal availability of various fresh or frozen fruits and vegetables.

During maintenance, keep an eye out for adverse psychological states like depression that might develop, and for evidence of binge eating. It is critical to deal with such problems early on.

Perhaps the most important tool for maintenance, though, is belief in your own ability to succeed. Self-talk is important during all stages of change. There is nothing inherently different about modifying your behaviors on Day 1 of your action stage than on Day 1000 of maintenance. Remind yourself that you have accomplished much already, and maintain your well-founded belief in your own ability to stay the course you have set for yourself. If you have followed the advice in this book, your goals are reasonable and so are the methods you have used to achieve and maintain them. They have also been carefully individualized by you to match your needs.

You have carefully assessed your motivations, your diet, your behaviors, and your level of physical activity, and you have incorporated each in your Personal Plan of Action. Rededicate yourself to your Personal Plan periodically, and watch your maintenance last and last. You deserve nothing less. Good luck!

Pyramid Food Tables for Weight Management and Pyramid Pattern Menus

Pyramid Food Tables for Weight Management

The following foods are classified according to the food groups depicted in the Food Guide Pyramid. Consequently, there is a bread, cereal, rice, and pasta table; a table of vegetables; a table of fruits; a milk, yogurt, and cheese table; and a table of meats and meat substitutes (which includes poultry, fish, dry beans, eggs, and nuts). You will also find additional tables for foods that do not fit neatly into the five major categories, either because they do not have enough key nutrients relative to calories, or because they have very little nutrient *and* caloric value, or because a food is actually a combination of two or more of the five nutrient-rich categories. These tables include fats, oils, and sweets; miscellaneous "free" foods; and combination foods. Finally, there are tables for fast foods and ethnic foods.

Within each table, foods are arranged in alphabetical order. In the five major food groups, every effort was made to indicate the usual, standard serving for each food. In a few cases, however, nutrient density principles dictated an unusually large amount as a serving. In order to avoid confusion, these inflated items were sometimes left in their group rather than moved to the fats, oils, and sweets group (pecans, which appear in the meat and meat substitutes group, are a good example).

For each food the number of fat grams and total calories is listed relative to the serving size or amount indicated. These amounts count as *one serving* (unless otherwise indicated) according to the nutrient density principles of the Food Guide Pyramid. In the fats, oils, and sweets table, servings may have been adjusted from the norm to comply with an arbitrary standard of 75–150 calories or an average of 115 calories per serving. Each of these foods, according to the amount listed, also counts as *one serving* when keeping track on Pyramid Monitoring Guides. In some cases, certain foods which would ordinarily be included in one of the five nutrient-rich food categories have been moved to the fats, oils, and sweets list to reflect a high calorie level relative to other nutrients due to the addition of fat, sugar, or both. We have taken the liberty of making these distinctions for the purposes of weight management. *These adjustments are clearly indicated.*

Within each of the five nutrient-rich groups, foods are divided into low or higher fat choices. Foods in **boldface type** represent a lower fat choice within the food group. Foods that are *both* in boldface and in *italic* are calorically exchangeable, both among themselves and with foods in the preplanned menus. Low-fat (boldface) foods are distinguished from higher fat choices according to the following fat gram per serving criteria: Bread, cereal, rice, and pasta group—1 or fewer; vegetable and fruit groups—1 or fewer; milk, yogurt, and cheese—1 or fewer; meat and meat substitutes—7 or fewer. Foods have also been put in boldface in the tables for combination foods, fast foods, and ethnic foods to reflect a lower fat choice (less than 30% of calories from fat). For weight management purposes you may carefully include the higher fat choices (those not in boldface) in all tables in the context of an entire day's intake with the recommended goal of keeping your fat consumption *less* than 30% (preferably 15–25%) of total calories.

Table of Contents

MEASUREMENT GUIDE—EQUIVALENTS

Volume

1 tablespoon = ½ fluid ounce = 3 teaspoons
¼ cup = 2 fluid ounces = 4 tablespoons
½ cup = 4 fluid ounces = 8 tablespoons
1 cup = 8 fluid ounces
2 cups = 1 pint
2 pints = 1 quart

Weight

1 ounce = 28 grams
4 ounces = ¼ pound
8 ounces = ½ pound
16 ounces = 1 pound

Guesstimates

3 ounces meat/fish/poultry = a deck of cards or a cassette tape
1 cup of potatoes/rice/pasta = a tennis ball
1 ounce of cheese = a pair of dice

MEAT AND MEAT SUBSTITUTES—EXAMPLES

One-ounce portions*	Two-ounce portions**	Three-ounce portions**
1 egg	2 eggs	3 eggs
1 oz cheese***	2 oz cheese***	3 oz cheese
¼ c egg substitute	½ c egg substitute	¾ c egg substitute
2 Tbsp peanut butter	4 Tbsp peanut butter	6 Tbsp peanut butter
¼ c cottage cheese	½ c cottage cheese	¾ c cottage cheese
⅛ c or 2 Tbsp tuna	¼ c tuna	⅓ c tuna
½ c beans	1 c beans	1½ c beans
1–2 slices lunch meat	1 small chicken leg or thigh	1 small chicken breast, pork chop, hamburger patty, or medium fish fillet

*Equivalent to ⅓–½ meat serving.
**Equivalent to 1 meat serving.
***May substitute up to 1–2 oz cheese for 1–2 oz meat per day.

EXPLANATION OF ABBREVIATIONS

Tbsp = tablespoon	lb = pound	w/ = with
tsp = teaspon	pkt = packet	c = cup
oz = ounce	w/o = without	

CONVERSIONS

rice:	1 c uncooked	= 3 c cooked
noodles:	1 c uncooked	= 1 c cooked
macaroni:	1 c uncooked	= 2½ c cooked
spaghetti:	8 oz uncooked	= 4 c cooked
popcorn:	¼ c unpopped	= 5 c popped
cheese:	4 oz	= 1 c shredded
	1 lb	= 4 c shredded

BREAD, CEREAL, RICE, AND PASTA
For Energy, Vitamins, Minerals, and Fiber

Food Item	Serving Size	Fat Grams	Calories
Bagel, frozen,*	**½ small**	**1**	**110**
Barley, cooked	**½ c**	**0**	**97**
Biscuit	1 small	4	95
Bread, Boboli	½ small	3	160
Bread, Boboli	⅛ of a large	3.5	150
Bread, light, white or wheat	*2 slices*	*1*	*80*
Bread, french, italian, *pumpernickel, or rye*	*1 slice*	*1*	*81*
Bread, sweet (banana nut, pumpkin, etc.)	1 oz	3	85
Bread, white, wheat, *sourdough, or potato*	*1 slice*	*1*	*70*
Cereal, hot (grits, oatmeal, *cream of wheat/rice)*	*½ c*	*0*	*70*
Cereal, ready-to-eat, **unsweetened**	**1 oz**	**0**	**110**
Cereal, ready-to-eat, **sweetened**	**1 oz**	**1**	**110**
Cornbread	2-oz piece	5	144
Corn tortilla	*1 (8")*	*1*	*67*
Couscous	**½ c**	**1**	**100**
Crackers, buttery-type (e.g. Ritz or Club)	8	8	140
Crackers, graham, plain	3, 3" squares	2	90
Crackers, melba rounds	*7*	*1*	*70*
Crackers, oyster	30	3	99
Crackers, saltines	8	3	96
Croissant	½ medium	8	125
Croutons	⅓ c	3	80
English muffin	*½*	*1*	*65*
French toast, frozen	1 slice	2	85
French toast, homemade	1 slice	7	153
Granola, w/ or w/o raisins	¼ c or 1 oz	5	130
Granola, low-fat	1 oz	1.5	105
Granola bar, crunchy	1	5	120
Granola bar, low-fat, chewy	1	2	110
Granola bar, chewy	1	5	130
Macaroni	**½ c**	**0**	**99**
Muffin (bran, blueberry, corn, apple, etc.)	1 mini, ¼ large, or 1 oz	3	100

BREAD, CEREAL, RICE, AND PASTA (Cont.)

Food Item	Serving Size	Fat Grams	Calories
Muffin, light	**1 small or 1½ oz**	1	111
Noodles, egg	**½ c**	1	106
Pancake	4"	2	69
Pasta, spaghetti	**½ c**	0	100
Pita pocket bread	**½ large** **or 1 medium**	1	110
Popcorn, air-popped, unbuttered	*4 c*	*1*	*80*
Popcorn, microwave, light	4 c	3	95
Popcorn, oil-popped, unbuttered	4 c	16	247
Pretzels, plain	**1 oz**	1	111
Pretzels, cheddar or cream caramel	1 oz	6.5	160
Pretzels, buttermilk ranch or honey mustard and onion	1 oz	5.5	130
Rice, brown	**½ c**	1	116
Rice cakes	*2 large or 10 mini*	*0*	*90*
Rice, white	**½ c**	0	110
Rice, wild	**½ c**	1	130
Roll, crescent, plain	1	6	100
Roll, dinner, pan, plain	1	2	85
Roll, hamburger	*½*	*1*	*60*
Roll, hard	*½*	*1*	*85*
Roll, hot dog	*½*	*1*	*60*
Tortilla, corn	*6"*	*1*	*67*
Tortilla, flour	8"	2	85
Waffle, plain	1 small	3	90

*A whole deli-size bagel counts as three servings.

VEGETABLES
For Vitamins, Minerals, and Fiber
(Prepared and eaten without added fat except where indicated)

Food Item	Serving Size	Fat Grams	Calories
Artichoke, boiled or steamed	**½ medium**	0	27
Artichoke hearts, steamed	**½ c**	0	37
Asparagus, canned	**½ c**	1	24
Asparagus, cooked	*½ c or 4 spears*	*0*	*19*
Beans, baked**	**½ c**	0.5	125
Beets, canned, harvard*	**½ c**	0	90
Beets, canned, pickled*	**½ c**	0	75
Broccoli, cooked	*½ c*	*0*	*23*

Food Item	Serving Size	Fat Grams	Calories
Broccoli, raw, chopped	½ c	0	12
Brussels sprouts	½ c	0	30
Cabbage, cooked	½ c	0	16
Cabbage, raw	1 c	0	16
Carrots, cooked	½ c	0	35
Carrots, raw	1 medium	0	31
Cauliflower, cooked	½ c	0	15
Cauliflower, raw, chopped	½ c	0	12
Celery, raw	1 stalk	0	6
Corn, canned*	½ c	1	66
Corn, cream style*	½ c	1	93
Corn on the cob*	1, 5" ear	1	70
Eggplant, raw or cooked	½ c	0	12
Green beans, cooked	½ c	0	22
Greens (kale, turnip, etc.), cooked	½ c	0	25
Legumes (beans), all types, cooked**	½ c	0	115
Lettuce, iceberg	1 c	0	8
Lettuce, leaf	1 c	0	10
Lettuce, romaine	1 c	0	8
Mixed vegetables (w/ corn, peas)*	½ c	0	55
Mushrooms, cooked	½ c	0	21
Mushrooms, raw, chopped	½ c	0	9
Onion, cooked	½ c	0	29
Onion, raw, chopped	½ c	0	27
Parsnips, boiled*	½ c	0	63
Peas, green, cooked*	½ c	0	67
Peppers, bell, cooked	½ c	0	12
Peppers, bell, raw, chopped	½ c	0	12
Potatoes, french-fried, frozen, heated*	10 strips	4	111
Potatoes, hash brown, homemade*	½ c	11	163
Potatoes, mashed, homemade*	½ c	4	111
Potatoes, O'Brien*	½ c	1	80
Potatoes, scalloped*	½ c	7	160
Potato, sweet or yam*	1 large	0	118
Potato, baked w/ skin*	1 medium	0	120
Pumpkin, boiled, mashed	½ c	0	24
Pumpkin, canned	½ c	0	41
Radishes, raw	10 pieces	0	7
Rhubarb, frozen, raw, chopped	½ c	0	15
Salad, three-bean*	⅓ c	0	95

VEGETABLES (Cont.)

Food Item	Serving Size	Fat Grams	Calories
Sauerkraut, canned	*½ c*	*0*	*22*
Spinach, cooked	*½ c*	*0*	*21*
Spinach, raw	*1 c*	*0*	*12*
Squash, acorn, cooked*	*½ c*	*0*	*50*
Squash, butternut	*½ c*	*0*	*45*
Squash, yellow, crookneck, cooked	*½ c*	*0*	*18*
Squash, yellow, crookneck, raw, chopped	*½ c*	*0*	*12*
Squash, zucchini, cooked	*½ c*	*0*	*14*
Squash, zucchini, raw, chopped	*½ c*	*0*	*9*
Tomato, canned	*½ c*	*0*	*30*
Tomato, fresh	*1 whole*	*0*	*23*
Tomato juice	*¾ c*	*0*	*36*
Tomato sauce	*½ c*	*0*	*40*

*Starchy vegetables: Because of their higher starch content, some of these choices are higher in calories per serving. Be sure to include some for variety, but try not to choose more than one serving per day **as a vegetable** to ensure that over time your average calories fall within your budget for weight loss. You may, however, opt to substitute these items for an occasional bread/starch serving.

**A starchy vegetable that can substitute for either a bread/starch serving or for 1 ounce of lean meat. See meat and meat substitutes list.

FRUIT
For Vitamins, Minerals, and Fiber

Food Item	Serving Size	Fat Grams	Calories
Apple	**1 medium**	**1**	**81**
Apple juice	**¾ c**	**0**	**95**
Applesauce, unsweetened	*½ c*	*0*	*53*
Apricots, dried	**8 halves**	**0**	**83**
Apricots, fresh	*4 medium*	*1*	*68*
Avocado, puréed	½ c	18	203
Avocado, sliced	½ medium	15	153
Banana	**1 medium**	**1**	**105**
Berries (strawberries, raspberries, blackberries, etc.)	*½ c*	*0*	*40*
Cantaloupe	*¼ whole (medium) or 1 c cubes*	*0*	*57*
Cherries, sweet, fresh	*12*	*1*	*59*
Cranberry juice cocktail	**¾ c**	**0**	**110**

Food Item	Serving Size	Fat Grams	Calories
Cranberry juice, light	*¾ c*	*0*	*30*
Dates, dried	*3, or*		
	2 Tbsp chopped	*0*	*68*
Figs, dried	2	0	95
Fruit cocktail, juice pack	*½ c*	*0*	*60*
Grapefruit	1	0	80
Grapefruit juice	¾ c	0	72
Grape juice	¾ c	0	106
Grapes	*1 c*	*0*	*60*
Honeydew	*¹⁄₁₀ whole (medium)*		
	or ½ c cubes	1	66
Kiwi	*1 large*	*0*	*46*
Mango	*½*	*0*	*68*
Nectarine	1 medium	0.5	70
Orange	1 medium	0	80
Orange juice	¾ c	0	78
Orange, mandarin, juice pack	*½ c*	*0*	*58*
Peach, fresh	*1 whole*	*0*	*40*
Peaches, canned, juice pack	*½ c*	*0*	*60*
Pear, canned, juice pack	*½ c*	*0*	*62*
Pear, fresh	1 whole	0	100
Pineapple, canned, juice pack	½ c cubes	0	75
Pineapple, fresh	*½ c*	*0*	*40*
Pineapple juice	¾ c	0	102
Plum	*1 medium*	*0*	*36*
Prune juice	*¾ c*	*0*	*135*
Prunes, dried	*3*	*0*	*60*
Raisins	*2 Tbsp*	*0*	*62*
Tangelo	*1*	*0*	*40*
Tangerine	*1 small*	*0*	*40*
Watermelon	*½ c cubes*	*0*	*25*

MILK, YOGURT, AND CHEESE
For Calcium and Protein

Food Item	Serving Size	Fat Grams	Calories
Cheese, Alpine Lace, american	2 oz	14	160
Cheese, Alpine Lace, swiss	2 oz	10	150
Cheese, american	2 oz	18	212
Cheese, american, fat-free	*2 oz*	*0*	*80*
Cheese, cheddar	1½ oz	14	171
Cheese, cheddar, fat-free	*1½ oz*	*0*	*67*

MILK, YOGURT, AND CHEESE (Cont.)

Food Item	Serving Size	Fat Grams	Calories
Cheese, cheddar, ⅓ less fat	1½ oz	7	120
Cheese, cottage, 1%	2 c	4	328
Cheese, cottage, 2%	2 c	8	406
Cheese, cottage, whole milk, 4%	2 c	20	434
Cheese, feta	2 oz	12	150
Cheese, monterey	1½ oz	13	159
Cheese, mozzarella, whole milk	2 oz	12	160
Cheese, mozzarella, fat-free	**1½ oz**	**0**	**67**
Cheese, mozzarella, part skim	1½ oz	8	108
Cheese, muenster	1½ oz	13	157
Cheese, parmesan, grated, canned	¼ c	6	92
Cheese, parmesan, grated, from hard	1 oz	7	111
Cheese, provolone	1½ oz	11	150
Cheese, ricotta, part skim	½ c	10	171
Cheese, ricotta, whole milk	½ c	16	216
Cheese, swiss	1½ oz	12	161
Ice milk*	1½ c	9	276
Milk, chocolate, 1%	1 c	4	158
Milk, chocolate, 2%	1 c	6	180
Milk, chocolate, whole	1 c	10	208
Milk, white, 1%	1 c	3	102
Milk, white, 2%	1 c	5	120
Milk, white, nonfat (skim)	**1 c**	**0**	**86**
Milk, white, whole, 3.3%	1 c	8	150
Milk, white, whole, 4%	1 c	10	170
Pudding, regular, made w/ skim milk	**1 c**	**0**	**264**
Pudding, regular, made w/ 2% milk	1 c	6	300
Pudding, regular, made w/ whole milk	1 c	8	324
Pudding, sugar-free, made w/ 2% milk	1 c	6	180
Pudding, sugar-free, made w/ skim milk	**1 c**	**0**	**145**
Yogurt, frozen, low-fat*	1½ c	12	354
Yogurt, frozen, nonfat*	**1½ c**	**0**	**339**
Yogurt, nonfat, flavored, made w/ non-nutritive sweetener	**1 c**	**0**	**100**

Food Item	Serving Size	Fat Grams	Calories
Yogurt, plain, or w/ non-nutritive sweetener made with 2% milkfat	1 c	4	125
Yogurt, plain, made w/ whole milk	1 c	8	140
Yogurt, plain, nonfat	**1 c**	**0**	**120**
Yogurt, sweetened, made w/ 1–2% milkfat	1 c	4	220
Yogurt, sweetened, made w/ whole milk	1 c	6	254
Yogurt, sweetened, nonfat	**1 c**	**0**	**150**

*These items must contain 15% daily value for calcium per ½ cup serving.

MEAT AND MEAT SUBSTITUTES*
Good Sources of Protein and Iron

Food Item	Serving Size	Fat Grams	Calories
Almonds, dry-roasted	2–3 oz	30–45	344–516
Beans, black	**1–1½ c**	**0**	**240–360**
Beans, kidney	**1–1½ c**	**0**	**226–339**
Beans, navy	**1–1½ c**	**2–3**	**258–387**
Beans, pinto, dried, cooked	**1–1½ c**	**0**	**236–354**
Beans, refried	**1–1½ c**	**4–6**	**270–405**
Beef, brisket	2–3 oz	15–22	200–300
Beef, corned	2–3 oz	11–16	143–215
Beef, ground, lean	2–3 oz	11–16	153–230
Beef, ground, regular	2–3 oz	11–17	165–248
Beef, ground, sirloin	2–3 oz	9–14	149–223
Beef, prime rib	2–3 oz	17–26	218–327
Beef roast, lean	2–3 oz	7–10	133–200
Beefsteak, filet, broiled	***2–3 oz***	***5–8***	***117–175***
Beefsteak, flank, broiled	2–3 oz	9–13	145–218
Beefsteak, porterhouse, broiled	2–3 oz	9–14	148–222
Beefsteak, sirloin, broiled	2–3 oz	7–11	139–209
Bologna, regular	4–6 oz	36–54	364–546
Bologna, turkey	4–6 oz	18–27	240–360
Canadian bacon	***3–5 oz***	***3–5***	***90–150***
Cashews	3–5 oz	39–65	489–815
Chicken breast, fried, w/ skin	**2–3 oz**	**5–8**	**124–187**
Chicken drumstick, fried, w/ skin	2–3 oz	8–12	141–212
Chicken thigh, fried, w/ skin	2–3 oz	8–12	147–221

MEAT AND MEAT SUBSTITUTES (Cont.)

Food Item	Serving Size	Fat Grams	Calories
Chicken, roasted, dark meat, w/o skin	*2–3 oz*	*6–9*	*117–176*
Chicken, roasted, white meat, w/o skin	*2–3 oz*	*3–4*	*99–148*
Chicken, roasted, w/ skin, light and dark	2–3 oz	8–12	137–205
Clams, breaded and fried	4 oz or 12 small	12	228
Clams, steamed	*2–3 oz or 19 small*	*1–2*	*84–126*
Crab cake, cooked w/ fat	1, 3 oz	8	152
Crab, cooked w/ moist heat	*2–3 oz*	*1–2*	*58–87*
Crab, imitation, surimi	*4–6 oz*	*2–3*	*116–174*
Egg, boiled, hard or soft	2–3 eggs	12–18	154–231
Egg, scrambled, w/ milk and fat	2–3 eggs	14–21	190–285
Egg substitute	*½–¾ c*	*0*	*60–90*
Egg white, hard-cooked	*1–3 eggs*	*0*	*23–48*
Fish, flounder	*2–3 oz*	*1*	*66–99*
Fish, flounder, stuffed w/ crabmeat filling	*2–3 oz*	*3–5*	*73–110*
Fish, orange roughy	*2–3 oz*	*1*	*50–75*
Fish, perch	*2–3 oz*	*1*	*66–99*
Fish, salmon	*2–3 oz*	*3–5*	*95–143*
Fish sticks	4–6 oz	14–20	304–456
Fish, tuna, steak	*2–3 oz*	*1*	*77–115*
Fish, tuna, canned in oil, dark	*2–3 oz*	*5–7*	*113–169*
Fish, tuna, canned in oil, white	*2–3 oz*	*5–7*	*105–158*
Fish, tuna, canned in water, dark	*2–3 oz*	*0–1*	*66–99*
Fish, tuna, canned in water, white	*2–3 oz*	*1–2*	*77–116*
Ham, canned or roasted, lean	2–3 oz	8–12	140–210
Hot dog, beef, 8 per 1-lb package	2–3 franks	32–48	360–540
Hot dog, chicken or turkey, 8 per 1-lb package	2–3 franks	18–27	232–348
Hot dog, pork, 8 per 1-lb package	2–3 franks	34–51	368–552
Lamb, rib or loin, lean, broiled or roasted	2–3 oz	7–10	133–195
Oysters, breaded and fried	6–9 oz or 12–15 medium	22–33	340–510
Oysters, raw	*6–9 oz*	*4–6*	*116–174*
Oysters, steamed	*4–6 oz or 16–24 medium*	*6–8*	*156–234*
Peanut butter	4–6 Tbsp	23–48	376–564

Food Item	Serving Size	Fat Grams	Calories
Peanuts	2–3 oz	28–42	328–492
Pecans	7–12 oz	133–228	1330–2280
Pepperoni	2–4 oz	24–48	270–540
Pork chop, broiled	2–3 oz	15–23	196–294
Pork chop, fried	2–3 oz	19–28	223–334
Pork, rump, lean, roasted	2–3 oz	7.5–11	126–189
Pork, shoulder, roasted	2–3 oz	10–14	147–163
Pork, spare ribs, braised	2–3 oz	18–26	227–340
Salami	4–6 oz	22–33	274–411
Sardines, canned in oil	5–7 or 2–3 oz	7–11	125–175
Sausage, italian, pork	1–2 links or 2½–5 oz	17–34	217–424
Sausage, link, breakfast	5–8 or 2½–4 oz	20–33	240–384
Sausage patty, ground	3–6 oz	25–50	300–600
Sausage, polish	3–6 oz	24–48	276–552
Sausage, turkey	*2–4 oz*	*5–10*	*90–180*
Scallops, broiled	*2–3 oz*	*0.5–1*	*100–150*
Shrimp, boiled	*2–3 oz*	*1*	*56–84*
Shrimp, breaded and fried	2–3 oz	7–10	137–206
Sunflower seeds, dry-roasted	2½–4 oz	35–56	412–660
Tofu, raw	¾–1 c	9–12	141–248
Turkey, dark meat, roasted, w/ skin	*2–3 oz*	*7–10*	*126–189*
Turkey, dark meat, roasted, w/o skin	*2–3 oz*	*4–6*	*107–160*
Turkey ham	*3–4 oz*	*4.5–6*	*105–140*
Turkey, white meat, roasted, w/ skin	*2–3 oz*	*5–7*	*113–169*
Turkey, white meat, roasted, w/o skin	*2–3 oz*	*4–6*	*90–135*
Veal, ground, broiled	*2–3 oz*	*5–7*	*98–147*
Veal, leg, roasted	*2–3 oz*	*3–4*	*91–137*
Veal, leg, pan-fried, breaded	*2–3 oz*	*3–5*	*130–195*
Veal, loin, lean and fat, roasted	2–3 oz	7–11	124–186
Veal, loin, lean only, roasted	*2–3 oz*	*4–6*	*100–150*
Veal, shoulder, lean, roasted	*2–3 oz*	*4–6*	*94–146*
Veal, sirloin, lean, roasted	*2–3 oz*	*3–5*	*96–144*
Veal, stew meat, lean	*2–3 oz*	*3–4*	*107–161*
Vegetable burger	1–1½	5–7.5	140–210
Walnuts	4–6 oz	76–114	760–1140

*All values given are for cooked portions if applicable.

FATS, OILS, AND SWEETS

(High in fat, sugar, or both relative to protein, vitamins, and minerals and/or traditionally considered to be desserts or snacks)

Food Item	Serving Size	Fat Grams	Calories
Alcohol, beer	12 oz	0	150
Alcohol, beer, light	12 oz	0	100
Alcohol, gin, 90 proof	1½ oz	0	110
Alcohol, liqueurs, coffee–type	1½ oz	0	165
Alcohol, rum, 80 proof	1½ oz	0	97
Alcohol, vodka, 80 proof	1½ oz	0	97
Alcohol, whiskey, 86 proof	1½ oz	0	105
Alcohol, wine, table, all types	3½ oz	0	72
Bacon	3 strips	9	108
Bacon pieces	4 Tbsp	4	100
Brownies w/ nuts, homemade*	1 small	6	97
Butter, stick	1 Tbsp	12	108
Cake, angel food*	2" slice or ¹⁄₁₂ of cake	0	150
Cake, carrot, iced*	1" by 1"	9	150
Cake, cheese, N.Y. style	¹⁄₃₂ cake (½ slice)	9	129
Cake, chocolate, iced, layer*	¹⁄₃₂ cake (½ slice)	6	117
Cake, iced, snack-type, fat-free*	1" by 1"	0	100
Cake, pound*	1" slice or ¹⁄₃₂ of cake	8	150
Cake, pound, fat-free*	1½" slice or ¹⁄₁₆ of cake	0	130
Cake, snack-type*	1" by 1"	4	100
Cake, vanilla, iced*	¹⁄₃₂ cake (½ slice)	6	150
Candy, bridge mix	1 oz	6	140
Candy corn	2 Tbsp	0	91
Candy, hard	1 oz	0	110
Candy, M&M's peanut	1 oz	7.5	144
Candy, M&M's plain	1 oz	6	136
Candy, milk chocolate	1 oz	10	150
Cheese, neufchâtel	2 Tbsp	7	74
Cheese spread**	1 oz	6	80
Chips, cheese curls	1 oz	11	150
Chips, corn	1 oz	9	150
Chips, potato	1 oz	10	150
Chips, tortilla	1 oz	8	150
Chocolate, hot, prep w/ water	1 c	1	120
Chocolate, hot, made w/ non-nutritive sweetener, prep w/ water	2 c	2	100

Food Item	Serving Size	Fat Grams	Calories
Cookie, animal*	14	3	120
Cookie, chocolate chip*	2 small	4	99
Cookie, fig newton*	2	2	120
Cookie, oatmeal*	2 small	5	124
Cookie, peanut butter*	2 small	5	110
Cookie, sandwich*	2	5	100
Cookie, shortbread*	2 small	4	84
Cookie, sugar*	3 small	5	107
Cream, half-and-half	3 Tbsp	6	75
Cream cheese, light	2 oz	10	124
Cream cheese, regular	1 oz	10	100
Cream, sour, light	¼ c	8	100
Cream, sour, regular	¼ c	12	120
Cream, whipping, heavy	2 Tbsp	12	104
Cupcake, cream-filled, iced, fat-free*	½ of 1 cake	0	80
Doughnut, cake-type	1	6	105
Doughnut, yeast, glazed	½ of 1 whole	8	135
Eclair	½ of 1 whole	7	119
Fruit punch	8 oz	0	120
Fruit roll up***	2	0	100
Fudgsicle	2	2	138
Gelatin, flavored	½ c	0	80
Gravy, canned	¾ c	6	90
Honey	2 Tbsp	0	128
Ice cream, premium**	¼ c	8	130
Ice cream, regular**	½ c	7	135
Ice cream sandwich	½ whole	6	120
Ice cream, soft-serve**	½ c	3	112
Jelly / preserves	2 Tbsp	0	100
Kool-aid / lemonade (frozen concentrate or powder)	8 oz	0	120
Lard	1 Tbsp	12	114
Margarine, light	2 Tbsp	12	102
Margarine, softspread, whipped	2 Tbsp	12	138
Margarine, regular, stick	1 Tbsp	12	102
Mayonnaise, light	2 Tbsp	12	100
Mayonnaise, regular	1 Tbsp	11	100
Oil (canola, corn, olive, peanut, sesame, or sunflower)	1 Tbsp	12	120
Olives, black	15 large	11	100
Olives, green	15 large	8	70
Pie, cream-type	1/16 of 9" pie	7	138

FATS, OILS, AND SWEETS (Cont.)

Food Item	Serving Size	Fat Grams	Calories
Pie, fruit, 2-crust	1/16 of 9" pie	6	140
Pie, pecan	1/32 of 9" pie	6	108
Pie, pumpkin	1/16 of 9" pie	7	121
Pie, snack, fried	1/4 of 1 large	5	100
Popsicles	2	0	100
Salad dressing, bleu cheese	1 Tbsp	8	77
Salad dressing, caesar	1 Tbsp	9	85
Salad dressing, light, all flavors	1/4 c	8	80
Salad dressing, italian or french	2 Tbsp	14	140
Salad dressing, ranch	2 Tbsp	10	120
Salad dressing, thousand island	2 Tbsp	12	120
Sherbet	1/2 c	2	135
Shortening, all vegetable	1 Tbsp	13	113
Soda, regular	6 oz	0	80
Sugar, brown	3 Tbsp	0	105
Sugar, white	2 Tbsp or 6 pkt	0	92
Sweet roll, cinnamon*	1/2 roll	4	79
Sweet roll, fruit*	1/2 roll	8	125
Syrup, chocolate	2 Tbsp	1	92
Syrup, maple and cane	2 Tbsp	0	100
Tea, sweetened, prep from instant powder	1 c or 8 oz	0	87
Toaster, pastry, plain or iced	1/2 of 1 whole	3	100
Whipped topping, Cool Whip	1/2 c	9	96
Whipped topping, Cool Whip Lite	1/2 c	8	72

*Placed in this group instead of bread, cereal, rice, and pasta group because of high sugar or high fat and sugar content relative to vitamins and minerals. If bread servings eaten for the day are too low compared to the recommended number of servings in your pyramid pattern and inclusion of these items will not inflate your total calories and fat grams above your daily budgets, you may consider this item as a bread serving.

**Placed in this group instead of milk group because of high sugar or high fat and sugar content relative to calcium. These are still good sources of calcium.

***Placed in this group instead of fruit group because of high added sugar content.

MISCELLANEOUS "FREE" FOODS
(Limit to 4 servings per day except those indicated—low in key nutrients and low in calories)

Food Item	Serving Size	Fat Grams	Calories
Au jus	2 oz or ¼ c	0	9
Broth, beef, bouillon	1 c	1	16
Broth, chicken	1 c	1	22
Catsup	1 Tbsp	0	17
Chewing gum, stick, regular or sugar-free	1 stick	0	8
Coffee	1 c	0	6
Cream cheese, fat-free	1 Tbsp or ½ oz	0	14
Cream, sour, fat-free	1 Tbsp	0	20
Crystal Light*	1 c or 8 oz	0	4
Gelatin, sugar-free*	½ c	0	8
Gravy, 98% fat-free, canned	2 oz or ¼ c	1	25
Horseradish	1 Tbsp	0	6
Kool-aid, sugar-free*	1 c	0	4
Margarine, soft spread, fat-free	1 tsp	0	5
Margarine, stick, fat-free	1 tsp	0	20
Mayonnaise, fat-free	1 Tbsp	0	16
Mustard, brown	1 Tbsp	1	15
Mustard, yellow	1 Tbsp	1	12
Picante sauce	¼ c	0	18
Pickles, bread and butter	2 slices	0	11
Pickles, dill	1 whole	0	7
Pickle relish	1 Tbsp	0	19
Salad dressing, fat-free, all flavors	1 Tbsp	0	12
Salsa	¼ c	0	20
Sauce, barbecue	1 Tbsp	0	15
Sauce, soy	1 Tbsp	0	10
Soda, diet*	12 oz	0	2
Tea, unsweetened*	1 c or 8 oz	0	3

*May have these foods/beverages in unlimited amounts.

COMBINATION FOODS (HOMESTYLE)*
(Represents 2 or more food groups)

Food Item	Serving Size	Fat Grams	Calories
Baked beans, w/ pork	½ c	**2**	**134**
Beef and vegetable stew	1 c	11	218
Chef salad (no dressing)	1½ c	16	267

COMBINATION FOODS (HOMESTYLE) (Cont.)

Food Item	Serving Size	Fat Grams	Calories
Chicken pot pie	⅓ of 9"	31	545
Chili (meat and beans)	1 c	9	268
Cole slaw, homemade	½ c	2	42
Grilled cheese w/ 1 oz of cheese	1	18	340
Lasagna (homemade) w/ meat	2½" by 4"	12	325
Macaroni and cheese	1 c	22	430
Meat loaf*	3 oz	10.5	150
Omelet, cheese	2 eggs	23	290
Pasta salad, creamy, store mix	½ c	10	200
Pasta salad, italian-style, store mix	½ c	6	150
Pizza (plain cheese)	**¼ of 12"**	**6**	**230**
Pizza, w/ pepperoni	¼ of 12"	9	250
Pizza, w/ sausage	¼ of 12"	10	270
Pizza, vegetable	**¼ of 12"**	**6**	**240**
Potato salad (homemade)	½ c	10	179
Quiche, w/ bacon	⅛ of pie	48	600
Quiche, spinach	⅛ of pie	16	220
Sandwich, BLT	1	16	290
Sandwich, bologna	1	16	305
Sandwich, chicken salad	1	20	355
Sandwich, club	1	26	570
Sandwich, egg salad	1	13	285
Sandwich, ham, plain	1	16	285
Sandwich, ham and cheese	1	24	390
Sandwich, ham salad	1	17	321
Sandwich, liverwurst, plain	1	12	260
Sandwich, peanut butter	1	20	385
Sandwich, peanut butter and jelly	1	15	350
Sandwich, roast beef, hot, w/ gravy	1	25	421
Sandwich, steak, sirloin	1	12	325
Sandwich, tuna salad	1	14	360
Sandwich, turkey, plain	**1**	**3**	**240**
Soup, beef noodle	1 c	3	84
Soup, beef vegetable	1 c	3	75
Soup, cheese, made w/ water	1 c	11	155
Soup, chicken noodle	1 c	3	83
Soup, chicken rice	1 c	2	60
Soup, clam chowder, manhattan	**1 c**	**2**	**78**
Soup, clam chowder, new england	1 c	7	163
Soup, cream of asparagus, broccoli, etc.	1 c	8	161

Food Item	Serving Size	Fat Grams	Calories
Soup, cream of chicken, crab, shrimp, etc.	1 c	9	180
Soup, minestrone	1 c	6	160
Soup, potato	**1 c**	**2**	**73**
Soup, tomato, made w/ milk	1 c	11	286
Soup, tomato, made w/ water	**1 c**	**2**	**86**
Soup, vegetable	**1 c**	**1**	**75**
Spaghetti w/ meat balls and tomato sauce	1 c	10	258
Spaghetti w/ meat sauce	**1 c**	**6**	**275**
Taco	1 small	9	182

*Homemade or ready-to-eat from grocery store.

FAST FOODS (GENERIC)
(Averaged from a number of chains in different locations)

Food Item	Serving Size	Fat Grams	Calories
Bacon cheeseburger	1 sandwich	27	464
Cheeseburger, regular	1 regular	15	299
Cheeseburger, large	1 large	32	524
Chicken, fried, dark meat	3 oz	15	234
Chicken, fried, light and dark meat	3 oz	14	235
Chicken, fried, light meat	3 oz	12	224
Chicken wings	5 wings	13	209
English muffin w/ egg, cheese, and bacon	1 sandwich	18	359
Fish, breaded and fried	1 portion	11	196
Fish sandwich	1 large sandwich	27	469
Fish sandwich, w/ cheese	1 regular sandwich	23	421
French fries	3 oz	14	274
Ham and cheese sandwich	1 sandwich	16	372
Hamburger, regular	1 regular	11	245
Hamburger, large	1 large	21	444
Hot dog	1 sandwich	14	214
Onion rings	3 oz	16	285
Pancakes w/ butter and syrup	**3 pancakes**	**10**	**468**
Pasta salad	¼ c	6	130
Pizza, cheese	**1 slice**	**9**	**290**

FAST FOODS (GENERIC) (Cont.)

Food Item	Serving Size	Fat Grams	Calories
Pizza, pepperoni	1 slice	12	306
Roast beef sandwich	1 regular	13	347
Shake	**10 fl oz**	**9**	**320**
Sundae	**1 regular**	**10**	**300**

THE "BEST" OF FAST FOODS*
(By specific restaurant)

Food Item	Serving Size	Fat Grams	Calories
ARBY'S			
Light roast beef deluxe	1	10	300
Light roast chicken deluxe	1	10	300
Light roast turkey deluxe	1	10	300
Roast beef junior	1	8.5	218
BURGER KING			
Breakfast bagel sandwich (plain)	1	14	387
Breakfast bagel sandwich (ham)	1	15	418
Chicken tenders	6 pieces	10	204
Chef salad (no dressing)	1	9	180
Chicken salad (no dressing)	**1**	**4**	**140**
Garden salad (no dressing)	1	5	90
Side salad (no dressing)	**1**	**0**	**20**
Reduced calorie italian dressing	1 Tbsp	2	30
Vanilla shake	**1**	**10**	**321**
CHICK-FIL-A			
Chargrilled chicken salad	**1**	**2**	**126**
Chargrilled chicken sandwich (reg and deluxe)	**1**	**5**	**258**
Chicken sandwich	**1**	**9**	**426**
Chicken deluxe sandwich	**1**	**9**	**435**
Chicken soup	**1 small**	**3**	**152**
Tossed salad (plain)	**1**	**0**	**21**
Lite italian dressing	**1 Tbsp**	**2**	**66**

Food Item	Serving Size	Fat Grams	Calories
DOMINO'S PIZZA			
Cheese pizza	**2 slices of a 16" large**	**10**	**376**
Sausage/mushroom pizza	2 slices of a 12" medium	16	430
HARDEE'S			
Pancakes (3) (no margarine or butter)	**1 order**	**2**	**280**
Pancakes (3) w/ 2 bacon strips	**1 order**	**9**	**350**
Pancakes (3) w/ 1 sausage patty	1 order	16	430
Roast beef sandwich	**1**	**9**	**260**
Hot ham and cheese sandwich	1	12	330
Chicken filet sandwich	1	13	370
Grilled chicken sandwich	1	9	310
Marinated grilled chicken sandwich	1	10	300
KFC			
Original recipe drumstick	1	8.5	146
Lite n' crispy drumstick	1	7	121
Cole slaw	1 order	6	114
Corn on the cob	**1**	**2**	**20**
Mashed potatoes w/ gravy	**1 order**	**2**	**71**
Apple bran muffin	**1**	**0**	**180**
McDONALD'S			
Egg McMuffin	1	11	280
Scrambled eggs	1	10	140
English muffin w/ butter	**1**	**6**	**170**
Hotcakes w/ 2 pats margarine and syrup	**1 order**	**12**	**435**
McGrilled chicken sandwich	**1**	**12**	**400**
McGrilled chicken classic sandwich	1	**3**	**250**
Hamburger, regular	1	9	225
Chicken fajita	1	8	185
Chunky chicken salad (no dressing)	1	**4**	**150**
French fries	1 small	12	220
Hash brown potatoes	1	7	130
Garden salad (no dressing)	1	2	50
Side salad (no dressing)	**1**	**1**	**30**
Lite vinaigrette dressing	1 Tbsp	2	48

Food Item	Serving Size	Fat Grams	Calories
McDONALD'S (Cont.)			
Red french low-cal dressing	1 Tbsp	8	160
Shakes (all)	1	5	**330**
Soft serve ice cream, vanilla			
low-fat frozen yogurt cone	1	1	**110**
Sundaes (all) w/o nuts	1	3	**240**
PIZZA HUT			
Cheese pizza, hand-tossed	1 slice	10	259
Cheese pizza, pan	1 slice of a medium	9	248
Cheese pizza, thin and crispy	1 slice of a medium	8.5	199
Pepperoni pizza, thin and crispy	1 slice of a medium	10	207
ROY ROGERS			
Pancake platter w/ syrup			
and butter	**1 order**	**15**	**452**
Pancake platter w/ bacon	1 order	18	493
Pancake platter w/ ham	**1 order**	**17**	**506**
Roast beef sandwich	1	10	317
Roast beef sandwich w/ cheese	1	12	**360**
Fried chicken drumstick	1	8	140
Cole slaw	1 order	7	110
Baked potato (plain)	1	1	**211**
Baked potato w/ margarine	1	7	**274**
Potato salad	1 order	6	107
Shakes (all)	1	10	**325**
Sundaes (caramel, strawberry)	1	8	**250**
TACO BELL			
Bean burrito	1	14	**447**
Border light bean burrito	1	6	**330**
Border light bean burrito supreme	1	8	**350**
Border light 7-layer burrito	1	9	**440**
Combination burrito	1	16	407
Border light taco	1	5	140
Border light taco supreme	1	5	**160**
Border light soft taco	1	5	**180**
Border light soft taco supreme	1	5	**200**
Chicken soft taco	1	10	213
Chicken fajita	1	10	226
Pintos and cheese	1	8.7	190

Food Item	Serving Size	Fat Grams	Calories
WENDY'S			
Toast w/ margarine	1 order	9	250
Grilled chicken sandwich	1	9	320
Jr. hamburger (2-oz kid's meal)	1	9	260
Chili	**8 oz**	8	**260**
Baked potato (plain)	1	2	**250**
Chili and cheese potato	1	18	500
Chicken a la king potato	1	6	**350**
Chef salad	1	5	130
Low-cal dressings	1 Tbsp	3	35

*All possible items for each restaurant *are not* listed. These foods were chosen to reflect the "best value," taking the following factors into consideration: total fat grams, total calories, satiety (how much it will fill you up), and whether these items can safely fit into a typical day's fat/calorie allowance for weight control. If a desired food is missing from the list, it is because the author felt that it was not a good weight management value.

ETHNIC FOODS

CHINESE			
Bamboo shoots	**¾ c**	**0**	**25**
Beef w/ broccoli	1 c	12	240
Beef chow mein	1 c	20	360
Chicken chow mein	1 c	16	320
Chop suey	1 c	10	203
Egg foo yung	1	20	265
Egg roll	1	10	225
Fortune cookie	**1**	**0**	**40**
Fried rice	½ c	10	170
Pepper steak	1 c	15	330
Sesame chicken	**1 c**	**12**	**400**
Shrimp chow mein	1 c	10	235
Shrimp egg foo yung w/ sauce	2 patties	31	367
Stir-fried vegetables	1 c	12	200
Sweet and sour chicken	**1 c**	**12**	**400**
Tofu	4 oz	5	75
Won ton soup	2 won tons	6	125

ITALIAN			
Eggplant parmigiana	4½ oz	25	353
Fettucine alfredo	5 oz	20	280

Food Item	Serving Size	Fat Grams	Calories
ITALIAN (Cont.)			
Lasagna (homemade) w/ meat	2½" by 4"	12	325
Linguini w/ clam sauce	10½ oz	10	290
Manicotti w/ marinara sauce	2 whole	17	365
Pizza (plain cheese)	**¼ of 12"**	**6**	**230**
Pizza, w/ pepperoni	¼ of 12"	9	250
Pizza, sausage	¼ of 12"	10	270
Pizza, vegetable	**¼ of 12"**	**6**	**240**
Ravioli w/ cheese	5 ravioli	15	263
Spaghetti w/ meat sauce	**1 c**	**6**	**275**
Spaghetti w/ meat balls and tomato sauce	1 c	10	258
JEWISH			
Borscht	**½ c**	**-**	**25**
Challah	**1 slice**	**1**	**80**
Herring, kippered or pickled	1 oz	3	55
Lox	1 oz	5	75
Matzo ball	1	6	125
Potato knish	2, 3" rounds	10	170
Potato latkes	½ c or 1, 4"	6	125
Smoked salmon	1 oz	5	75
MEXICAN			
Bean burrito	1 small, 7"	13	340
Bean dip	**2 Tbsp**	**-**	**60**
Beef burrito	**1 small, 9"**	**9**	**435**
Chili w/ beans	1 c	14	295
Chili w/o beans	1 c	23	345
Chimichanga, beef	5 oz	17	326
Corn chips	1 c	10	170
Enchilada, meat or cheese	1 small, 6"	13	325
Guacamole	2 Tbsp	5	45
Nachos, chips w/ cheese	3 oz	12	190
Picante sauce	**2 Tbsp**	**1**	**8**
Refried beans	½ c	15	255
Salsa	**2 Tbsp**	**-**	**10**
Spanish rice	½ c	8	187
Taco, beef	1	13	237
Taco salad	1 serving	19	430
Tamale w/ sauce	**1 large**	**8**	**272**
Tortilla chips	1 oz	7	140

Food Item	Serving Size	Fat Grams	Calories
Tostada, beans	**1 small**	**6**	**205**
Tostada, beef	1 small	10	200

Food values in these lists come from the following sources:
1. *Bowes and Church's Food Values of Portions Commonly Used,* by Jean A. T. Pennington, 15th ed. (1989); 16th ed. (1994).
2. *The Complete and Up-to-Date Fat Book,* by Karen J. Bellerson (1993).
3. *Eat for Health Food Guide,* by Giant Food, Inc. (1996).
4. *Environmental Nutrition,* vol. 18, no. 6 (June 1995).
5. *Healthy Dividends: A Plan for Balancing Your Fat Budget,* by the National Dairy Council (1990).
6. *Nutrition Facts:* actual product labels (1994).
7. *Nutritive Value of American Foods.* Agricultural Handbook No. 456, by the Agricultural Research Service, U.S. Department of Agriculture (1963).
8. *Tufts University Diet and Nutrition Letter,* vol. 12, no. 12 (February 1995).
9. *Tufts University Diet and Nutrition Letter,* vol. 13, no. 2 (April 1995).

Pyramid Pattern Menus

Key Points

- Bold items are the lowest calorie items in each category. Choose these items at least half the time to ensure that *over time* average calories fall in your daily plan's calorie range.
- If a category indicates that you may "choose 2," you may choose either 2 different items or *double* the amount of one item.
- You *may* alter the distribution of your food allowances. Each menu is just a sample. If you choose to re-arrange the order, just be careful not to add or delete allowed servings from the day.
- You may use the appropriate menu along with your food records to preplan your daily or weekly meals.
- By preplanning several days, you can do a better job of grocery shopping for exactly what you'll need.

Daily Eating Plans and Eating Patterns
1200–1400 Calories

DAILY EATING PLAN

Food Group	Number of Servings	Average Calories per Serving	Fat Grams per Serving
Bread/Cereal/Grain/Pasta (B)	6	90	0–3
Vegetables (V)	3	37	0
Fruits (F)	2	76	0
Milk and Milk Products (MK)	2	105	0–8
Meat and Meat Substitutes (MT)	2	126	0–10
Fats, Oils, and Sweets (FOS)	0–1	54	0–8

DAILY EATING PATTERN

Food Group	Breakfast	Lunch	Snack	Dinner
B	1	2	1	2
V		1		2
F	1	1		
MK	1		1	
MT		1		1
FOS	0–1			0–1

1400–1600 Calories

DAILY EATING PLAN

Food Group	Number of Servings	Average Calories per Serving	Fat Grams per Serving
Bread/Cereal/Grain/Pasta (B)	7	90	0–3
Vegetables (V)	4	37	0
Fruits (F)	2	76	0
Milk and Milk Products (MK)	2	105	0–8
Meat and Meat Substitutes (MT)	2	126	0–10
Fats, Oils, and Sweets (FOS)	0–2	54	0–8

DAILY EATING PATTERN

Food Group	Breakfast	Lunch	Snack	Dinner
B	2	2	1	2
V		2		2
F	1	1		
MK	1		1	
MT		1		1
FOS	0–2			0–2

1600–1800 Calories

DAILY EATING PLAN

Food Group	Number of Servings	Average Calories per Serving	Fat Grams per Serving
Bread/Cereal/Grain/Pasta (B)	8	90	0–3
Vegetables (V)	4	37	0
Fruits (F)	3	76	0
Milk and Milk Products (MK)	2	105	0–8
Meat and Meat Substitutes (MT)	2	126	0–10
Fats, Oils, and Sweets (FOS)	1–2	54	0–8

DAILY EATING PATTERN

Food Group	Breakfast	Lunch	Snack	Dinner
B	2	2	2	2
V		2		2
F	1	1	1	
MK	1		1	
MT		1		1
FOS	1–2			1–2

1800–2000 Calories

DAILY EATING PLAN

Food Group	Number of Servings	Average Calories per Serving	Fat Grams per Serving
Bread/Cereal/Grain/Pasta (B)	9	90	0–3
Vegetables (V)	5	37	0
Fruits (F)	3	76	0
Milk and Milk Products (MK)	2	105	0–8
Meat and Meat Substitutes (MT)	2	126	0–10
Fats, Oils, and Sweets (FOS)	1–3	54	0–8

DAILY EATING PATTERN

Food Group	Breakfast	Lunch	Snack	Dinner
B	3	2	2	2
V		2		3
F	1	1	1	
MK	1			1
MT		1		1
FOS	1–3		1–3	

2000–2200 Calories

DAILY EATING PLAN

Food Group	Number of Servings	Average Calories per Serving	Fat Grams per Serving
Bread/Cereal/Grain/Pasta (B)	10	90	0–3
Vegetables (V)	5	37	0
Fruits (F)	4	76	0
Milk and Milk Products (MK)	2	105	0–8
Meat and Meat Substitutes (MT)	2	126	0–10
Fats, Oils, and Sweets (FOS)	2–3	54	0–8

DAILY EATING PATTERN

Food Group	Breakfast	Lunch	Snack	Dinner
B	3	2	2	3
V		2		3
F	2	1	1	
MK	1			1
MT		1		1
FOS	2–3		2–3	

PYRAMID PATTERN MENU (1200–1400 CALORIES; 20–33 GRAMS OF FAT)

BREAKFAST	LUNCH
Bread Group, Choose 1	Bread Group, Choose 2
1 oz dry cereal	**1 slice bread**
½ small bagel	½ small bagel
½ english muffin	**7 melba rounds**
½ c cooked cereal	**½ english muffin**
1 slice toast	½ c pasta**
1 small muffin, light	½ c rice**
	½ hard roll
Fruit Group, Choose 1	Vegetable Group, Choose 1
¾ c 100% juice (GF, OJ)	1 med carrot
1 med banana	**1 c leafy greens**
1 med apple	1 med baked potato**
½ c honeydew	**1 whole tomato**
¼ med cantaloupe	½ c tomato sauce
2 Tbsp raisins	¾ c tomato juice
1 med orange	**½ c cooked vegetables (broccoli, asparagus, cauliflower,** greens**)**
1 med grapefruit	
Milk Group, Choose 1	Fruit Group, Choose 1
1 c skim milk	¾ c 100% juice (GF, OJ)
1½–2 oz fat-free cheese	1 med banana
1 c unsweetened or artificially sweetened nonfat yogurt	1 med apple
1½ oz reduced-fat cheese	**½ c honeydew**
1 c 1% milk	**¼ med cantaloupe**
1 c yogurt, nonfat	**2 Tbsp raisins**
	1 med orange
	1 med grapefruit
Fats, Oils, Sweets, Choose 0–1	Meat Group, Choose 1
1 Tbsp margarine***	**2–3 oz roasted turkey***
2 Tbsp jelly/preserves	**2–3 oz roasted chicken***
2 Tbsp syrup	**3–5 oz canadian bacon**
	½–¾ c egg substitute
	1–1½ c canned or cooked beans
	2–3 oz crab, tuna, or broiled fish
	2–3 oz broiled beef, steak, **filet**

* Skinless, white meat.

**Confine to no more than 1 time per day.

***Reduced-fat varieties are acceptable. Use fat-free varieties for additional servings.

SNACK	DINNER
Bread Group, Choose 1	**Bread Group, Choose 2**
½ small bagel	**1 slice bread**
4 c air-popped plain popcorn	½ small bagel
1 oz pretzels	**7 melba rounds**
2 large rice cakes	**½ english muffin**
1 oz dry cereal	½ c pasta**
7 melba rounds	½ c rice**
	½ hard roll
Milk Group, Choose 1	**Vegetable Group, Choose 2**
1 c skim milk	1 med carrot
1½–2 oz fat-free cheese	**1 c leafy greens**
1 c unsweetened or	1 med baked potato**
artificially sweetened	**1 whole tomato**
nonfat yogurt	½ c tomato sauce
1 c sugar-free pudding, made	¾ c tomato juice
with skim milk	**½ c cooked vegetables (broccoli,**
1 c 1% milk	**asparagus, cauliflower,** greens**)**
	Meat Group, Choose 1
	2–3 oz roasted turkey*
	2–3 oz roasted chicken*
	3–5 oz canadian bacon
	½–¾ c egg substitute
	1–1½ c canned or cooked beans
	2–3 oz crab, tuna, or broiled fish
	2–3 oz broiled beef, steak, **filet**
	Fats, Oils, Sweets, Choose 0–1
	1 Tbsp oil (vegetable, canola, olive)
	1 Tbsp margarine***
	15 olives
	1 Tbsp prepared regular
	salad dressing
	¼ c light salad dressing***
	1 Tbsp mayonnaise***

PYRAMID PATTERN MENU
(1400–1600 CALORIES; 23–39 GRAMS OF FAT)

BREAKFAST	LUNCH
Bread Group, Choose 2	**Bread Group, Choose 2**
1 oz dry cereal	**1 slice bread**
½ small bagel	½ small bagel
½ english muffin	**7 melba rounds**
½ c cooked cereal	**½ english muffin**
1 slice toast	½ c pasta**
1 small muffin, light	½ c rice**
	½ hard roll
Fruit Group, Choose 1	**Vegetable Group, Choose 2**
¾ c 100% juice (GF, OJ)	1 med carrot
1 med banana	**1 c leafy greens**
1 med apple	1 med baked potato**
½ c honeydew	**1 whole tomato**
¼ med cantaloupe	½ c tomato sauce
2 Tbsp raisins	¾ c tomato juice
1 med orange	**½ c cooked vegetables (broccoli,**
1 med grapefruit	**asparagus, cauliflower,** greens)
Milk Group, Choose 1	**Fruit Group, Choose 1**
1 c skim milk	¾ c 100% juice (GF, OJ)
1½–2 oz fat-free cheese	1 med banana
1 c unsweetened or	1 med apple
artificially sweetened	½ c honeydew
nonfat yogurt	**¼ med cantaloupe**
1½ oz reduced-fat cheese	**2 Tbsp raisins**
1 c 1% milk	1 med orange
1 c yogurt, nonfat	1 med grapefruit
Fats, Oils, Sweets, Choose 0–2	**Meat Group, Choose 1**
1 Tbsp margarine***	**2–3 oz roasted turkey***
2 Tbsp jelly/preserves	**2–3 oz roasted chicken***
2 Tbsp syrup	**3–5 oz canadian bacon**
	½–¾ c egg substitute
	1–1½ c canned or cooked beans
	2–3 oz crab, tuna, or broiled fish
	2–3 oz broiled beef, steak, **filet**

* Skinless, white meat.
**Confine to no more than 1 time per day.
***Reduced-fat varieties are acceptable. Use fat-free varieties for additional servings.

SNACK	DINNER
Bread Group, Choose 1	**Bread Group, Choose 2**
½ small bagel **4 c air-popped plain popcorn** 1 oz pretzels **2 large rice cakes** 1 oz dry cereal **7 melba rounds**	**1 slice bread** **½ small bagel** **7 melba rounds** **½ english muffin** ½ c pasta** ½ c rice** **½ hard roll**
Milk Group, Choose 1	Vegetable Group, Choose 2

1 c skim milk
1½–2 oz fat-free cheese
1 c unsweetened or
   artificially sweetened
   nonfat yogurt
1 c sugar-free pudding, made
   with skim milk
1 c 1% milk
	1 med carrot
	1 c leafy greens
	1 med baked potato**
	1 whole tomato
	½ c tomato sauce
	¾ c tomato juice
	**½ c cooked vegetables (broccoli,
	   asparagus, cauliflower,** greens**)**

	Meat Group, Choose 1
	2–3 oz roasted turkey* **2–3 oz roasted chicken*** **3–5 oz canadian bacon** **½–¾ c egg substitute** 1–1½ c canned or cooked beans **2–3 oz crab, tuna, or broiled fish** 2–3 oz broiled beef, steak, **filet**
	Fats, Oils, Sweets, Choose 0–2
	1 Tbsp oil (vegetable, canola, olive) 1 Tbsp margarine*** 15 olives 1 Tbsp prepared regular salad dressing ¼ c light salad dressing*** 1 Tbsp mayonnaise***

PYRAMID PATTERN MENU
(1600–1800 CALORIES; 27–44 GRAMS OF FAT)

BREAKFAST	LUNCH
Bread Group, Choose 2	**Bread Group, Choose 2**
1 oz dry cereal	**1 slice bread**
½ small bagel	½ small bagel
½ english muffin	**7 melba rounds**
½ c cooked cereal	**½ english muffin**
1 slice toast	½ c pasta**
1 small muffin, light	½ c rice**
	½ hard roll
Fruit Group, Choose 1	**Vegetable Group, Choose 2**
¾ c 100% juice (GF, OJ)	1 med carrot
1 med banana	**1 c leafy greens**
1 med apple	1 med baked potato**
½ c honeydew	**1 whole tomato**
¼ med cantaloupe	½ c tomato sauce
2 Tbsp raisins	¾ c tomato juice
1 med orange	**½ c cooked vegetables (broccoli,**
1 med grapefruit	**asparagus, cauliflower**, greens)
Milk Group, Choose 1	**Fruit Group, Choose 1**
1 c skim milk	¾ c 100% juice (GF, OJ)
1½–2 oz fat-free cheese	1 med banana
1 c unsweetened or	1 med apple
artificially sweetened	½ c honeydew
nonfat yogurt	¼ med cantaloupe
1½ oz reduced-fat cheese	**2 Tbsp raisins**
1 c 1% milk	1 med orange
1 c yogurt, nonfat	1 med grapefruit
Fats, Oils, Sweets, Choose 1–2	**Meat Group, Choose 1**
1 Tbsp margarine***	**2–3 oz roasted turkey***
2 Tbsp jelly/preserves	**2–3 oz roasted chicken***
2 Tbsp syrup	**3–5 oz canadian bacon**
	½–¾ c egg substitute
	1–1½ c canned or cooked beans
	2–3 oz crab, tuna, or broiled fish
	2–3 oz broiled beef, steak, **filet**

* Skinless, white meat.
**Confine to no more than 1 time per day.
***Reduced-fat varieties are acceptable. Use fat-free varieties for additional servings.

SNACK	DINNER
Bread Group, Choose 2	**Bread Group, Choose 2**
½ small bagel	**1 slice bread**
4 c air-popped plain popcorn	½ small bagel
1 oz pretzels	**7 melba rounds**
2 large rice cakes	**½ english muffin**
1 oz dry cereal	½ c pasta**
7 melba rounds	½ c rice**
	½ hard roll
Fruit Group, Choose 1	**Vegetable Group, Choose 2**
¾ c 100% juice (GF, OJ)	1 med carrot
1 med banana	**1 c leafy greens**
1 med apple	1 med baked potato**
½ c honeydew	**1 whole tomato**
¼ med cantaloupe	½ c tomato sauce
2 Tbsp raisins	¾ c tomato juice
1 med orange	**½ c cooked vegetables (broccoli,**
1 med grapefruit	**asparagus, cauliflower,** greens)
Milk Group, Choose 1	**Meat Group, Choose 1**
1 c skim milk	**2–3 oz roasted turkey***
1½–2 oz fat-free cheese	**2–3 oz roasted chicken***
1 c unsweetened or	**3–5 oz canadian bacon**
artificially sweetened	**½–¾ c egg substitute**
nonfat yogurt	1–1½ c canned or cooked beans
1 c sugar-free pudding, made	**2–3 oz crab, tuna, or broiled fish**
with skim milk	2–3 oz broiled beef, steak, **filet**
1 c 1% milk	
	Fats, Oils, Sweets, Choose 1–2
	1 Tbsp oil (vegetable, canola, olive)
	1 Tbsp margarine***
	15 olives
	1 Tbsp prepared regular
	salad dressing
	¼ c light salad dressing***
	1 Tbsp mayonnaise***

PYRAMID PATTERN MENU
(1800–2000 CALORIES; 30–50 GRAMS OF FAT)

BREAKFAST	LUNCH
Bread Group, Choose 3	**Bread Group, Choose 2**
1 oz dry cereal	**1 slice bread**
½ small bagel	**½ small bagel**
½ english muffin	**7 melba rounds**
½ c cooked cereal	**½ english muffin**
1 slice toast	½ c pasta**
1 small muffin, light	½ c rice**
	½ hard roll
Fruit Group, Choose 1	**Vegetable Group, Choose 2**
¾ c 100% juice (GF, OJ)	1 med carrot
1 med banana	**1 c leafy greens**
1 med apple	1 med baked potato**
½ c honeydew	**1 whole tomato**
¼ med cantaloupe	½ c tomato sauce
2 Tbsp raisins	¾ c tomato juice
1 med orange	**½ c cooked vegetables (broccoli,**
1 med grapefruit	**asparagus, cauliflower,** greens)
Milk Group, Choose 1	**Fruit Group, Choose 1**
1 c skim milk	¾ c 100% juice (GF, OJ)
1½–2 oz fat-free cheese	1 med banana
1 c unsweetened or	1 med apple
artificially sweetened	½ c honeydew
nonfat yogurt	**¼ med cantaloupe**
1½ oz reduced-fat cheese	**2 Tbsp raisins**
1 c 1% milk	1 med orange
1 c yogurt, nonfat	1 med grapefruit
Fats, Oils, Sweets, Choose 1–3	**Meat Group, Choose 1**
1 Tbsp margarine***	**2–3 oz roasted turkey***
2 Tbsp jelly/preserves	**2–3 oz roasted chicken***
2 Tbsp syrup	**3–5 oz canadian bacon**
	½–¾ c egg substitute
	1–1½ c canned or cooked beans
	2–3 oz crab, tuna, or broiled fish
	2–3 oz broiled beef, steak, **filet**

* Skinless, white meat.
**Confine to no more than 1 time per day.
***Reduced-fat varieties are acceptable. Use fat-free varieties for additional servings.

SNACK	DINNER
Bread Group, Choose 2	**Bread Group, Choose 2**
½ small bagel	**1 slice bread**
4 c air-popped plain popcorn	½ small bagel
1 oz pretzels	**7 melba rounds**
2 large rice cakes	**½ english muffin**
1 oz dry cereal	½ c pasta**
7 melba rounds	½ c rice**
	½ hard roll
Fruit Group, Choose 1	**Vegetable Group, Choose 3**
¾ c 100% juice (GF, OJ)	1 med carrot
1 med banana	**1 c leafy greens**
1 med apple	1 med baked potato**
½ c honeydew	**1 whole tomato**
¼ med cantaloupe	½ c tomato sauce
2 Tbsp raisins	¾ c tomato juice
1 med orange	**½ c cooked vegetables (broccoli,**
1 med grapefruit	**asparagus, cauliflower,** greens)
Fats, Oils, Sweets, Choose 1–3	**Milk Group, Choose 1**
1 Tbsp oil (vegetable, canola, olive)	**1 c skim milk**
1 Tbsp margarine***	**1½–2 oz fat-free cheese**
15 olives	**1 c unsweetened or**
1 Tbsp prepared regular	**artificially sweetened**
salad dressing	**nonfat yogurt**
¼ c light salad dressing***	1 c sugar free pudding, made with
1 Tbsp mayonnaise***	skim milk
	1 c 1% milk
	Meat Group, Choose 1
	2–3 oz roasted turkey*
	2–3 oz roasted chicken*
	3–5 oz canadian bacon
	½–¾ c egg substitute
	1–1½ c canned or cooked beans
	2–3 oz crab, tuna, or broiled fish
	2–3 oz broiled beef, steak, filet

PYRAMID PATTERN MENU
(2000–2200 CALORIES; 33–56 GRAMS OF FAT)

BREAKFAST	LUNCH
Bread Group, Choose 3	**Bread Group, Choose 2**
1 oz dry cereal	**1 slice bread**
½ small bagel	½ small bagel
½ english muffin	**7 melba rounds**
½ c cooked cereal	**½ english muffin**
1 slice toast	½ c pasta**
1 small muffin, light	½ c rice**
	½ hard roll
Fruit Group, Choose 2	**Vegetable Group, Choose 2**
¾ c 100% juice (GF, OJ)	1 med carrot
1 med banana	**1 c leafy greens**
1 med apple	1 med baked potato**
½ c honeydew	**1 whole tomato**
¼ med cantaloupe	½ c tomato sauce
2 Tbsp raisins	¾ c tomato juice
1 med orange	**½ c cooked vegetables (broccoli,**
1 med grapefruit	**asparagus, cauliflower,** greens)
Milk Group, Choose 1	**Fruit Group, Choose 1**
1 c skim milk	¾ c 100% juice (GF, OJ)
1½–2 oz fat-free cheese	1 med banana
1 c unsweetened or	1 med apple
artificially sweetened	**½ c honeydew**
nonfat yogurt	**¼ med cantaloupe**
1½ oz reduced-fat cheese	**2 Tbsp raisins**
1 c 1% milk	1 med orange
1 c yogurt, nonfat	1 med grapefruit
Fats, Oils, Sweets, Choose 2–3	**Meat Group, Choose 1**
1 Tbsp margarine***	**2–3 oz roasted turkey***
2 Tbsp jelly/preserves	**2–3 oz roasted chicken***
2 Tbsp syrup	**3–5 oz canadian bacon**
	½–¾ c egg substitute
	1–1½ c canned or cooked beans
	2–3 oz crab, tuna, or broiled fish
	2–3 oz broiled beef, steak, **filet**

* Skinless, white meat.
**Confine to no more than 1 time per day.
***Reduced-fat varieties are acceptable. Use fat-free varieties for additional servings.

SNACK	DINNER
Bread Group, Choose 2	**Bread Group, Choose 3**
½ small bagel	**1 slice bread**
4 c air-popped plain popcorn	½ small bagel
1 oz pretzels	**7 melba rounds**
2 large rice cakes	**½ english muffin**
1 oz dry cereal	**½ c pasta****
7 melba rounds	**½ c rice****
	½ hard roll
Fruit Group, Choose 1	Vegetable Group, Choose 3
¾ c 100% juice (GF, OJ)	1 med carrot
1 med banana	**1 c leafy greens**
1 med apple	1 med baked potato**
½ c honeydew	**1 whole tomato**
¼ med cantaloupe	½ c tomato sauce
2 Tbsp raisins	¾ c tomato juice
1 med orange	**½ c cooked vegetables (broccoli,**
1 med grapefruit	**asparagus, cauliflower,** greens**)**
Fats, Oils, Sweets, Choose 2–3	Milk Group, Choose 1
1 Tbsp oil (vegetable, canola, olive)	**1 c skim milk**
1 Tbsp margarine***	**1½–2 oz fat-free cheese**
15 olives	**1 c unsweetened or artificially**
1 Tbsp prepared regular	**sweetened nonfat yogurt**
salad dressing	1 c sugar free pudding, made with
¼ c light salad dressing***	skim milk
1 Tbsp mayonnaise***	1 c yogurt, nonfat
	1 c 1% milk
	Meat Group, Choose 1
	2–3 oz roasted turkey*
	2–3 oz roasted chicken*
	3–5 oz canadian bacon
	½–¾ c egg substitute
	1–1½ c canned or cooked beans
	2–3 oz crab, tuna, or broiled fish
	2–3 oz broiled beef, steak, **filet**

Index

Library of Congress Cataloging-in-Publication Data

Cheskin, Lawrence J.
  Losing weight for good : developing your personal plan of action / Lawrence
J. Cheskin.
    p.   cm.
Includes index.
ISBN 0-8018-5499-7 (alk. paper)
      1. Weight loss.   I. Title.
RM222.2.C474   1997   96-31948
613.2'5—dc20   CIP